ANXIE

TRAUMA

Guided Meditation to Healing Anxiety, Depression & Panic. Self Help Guide to Stress Relief. Sleep to Calm the Mind & Overcome the Trauma.

by

DAVID WARD

TABLE CONTENTS

INTRODUCTION 7
SIGNS OF TRAUMA 13

1. Anxiety or fear 13
2. Advancements of thoughts 13
3. Being startled by loud noises 14
4. Flashback of bad images 14
5. Physical symptoms 15
6. Lack of interest in usual activities 15
7. Sleep problems 16
8. Problems with thinking or concentration 16
9. Preoccupation with thinking about trauma 17
10. Guilt or self-doubt 17

PARTS OF THE BRAIN THAT ARE AFFECTED BY THE TRAUMA 18

Risk factors for PTSD 21

HOW PAIN, STRESS AND ANXIETY AFFECTS YOUR LIFE 26

How pain affects your life 26
How Stress and Anxiety Affects Your body and Life 30

HOW TO DEAL WITH TRAUMA 34

1. Safety first 34
2. Talking with someone you trust 34
4. Accepting the belief 35
5. You have to spend time doing relaxing things ... 35
6. Confronting the situations in an effective and disciplined manner 36
8. Education to the patients 37

COMPLEX PTSD BEHAVIOR AND HOW TO CONTROL IT 39

Complex PTSD: Beyond Trauma............................ 39
Behavior behind complex PTSD............................ 39
How to maintain control over yourself 41

COGNITIVE BEHAVIORAL THERAPY TOOLS FOR ANXIETY... 43

Mindfulness 44
Five Senses.. 47
Finding Colors 49
Muscle Relaxation 51

HOW TO USE TAPPING TO REDUCE PTSD 53

A Biological and Emotional Perspective 53
An Energetic Perspective...................................... 54
Trauma in the Chakras 54
Trauma and Addiction.. 55
How to Create Safety: Resourcing......................... 56
Guided Meditation.. 58

THE DISTRACTOR DISPUTING.................. 59

Behavioral Exercises... 60
Anxiety and trauma 61
Metacognitive Techniques.................................... 62
Metacognition helps in:.. 63

THE BENEFITS OF VAGUS NERVE STIMULATION 73

What is High Vagal Tone? 74
What is Low Vagal Tone? 76
How to Measure Vagal Tone 77
The Effects of Vagus Nerve Stimulation 79

ADRENALINE ADDICTION AND HIGH-RISK BEHAVIOR 82

ADRENALINE RUSH..84
ADRENALINE ADDICTION TEST 91

CHANGING MALADAPTIVE THINKING..... 99

The Main Goal Of Cognitive Behavioral Therapy ..99
Effective Considerations For The Assessment..... 101
Intervention & Treatment Analysis......................104
The Power Of CBT: Removal Of Erroneous Thinking 107

FACING YOUR FEARS 109

HEALING EXERCISES FOR BETTER SOCIAL FUNCTIONING 115

Anxiety, Social Situations, and the Vagus Nerve ..121

CONCLUSION 125

INTRODUCTION

Anxiety can take on many forms and can affect people in multiple ways. Sometimes people have generalized anxiety disorder and other people have anxieties that occur in very special circumstances. In this chapter, we will discuss the definition of anxiety, as well as the various ways that different people may be affected.

What is Anxiety?

There are two ways of looking at anxiety. One is the dictionary definition, which has most likely affected everyone in the world at some point in their lives. This view of anxiety describes it as nervousness, a worrying sensation, or not feeling at ease. This definition of anxiety typically concerns an event which a person may be uncertain how it will unfold or even about a specific looming event. This is the type of anxiety a person might feel just before giving an important presentation. This varies quite a bit from the clinical definition of anxiety as a mental disorder.

In the case, that anxiety is defined as a nervous disorder, the characteristics of which are classic feelings of unease in an excessive amount. It can also be described as an apprehension. In the majority of cases of anxiety, co morbidity exists of panic attacks or compulsive behaviors. This is the type of anxiety that can be debilitating to a person especially when combined with behavioral compulsions can come to rule over a person's life. For the purpose of this book, we will be referring to this definition of anxiety.

Anxiety can be very difficult to diagnose. Nearly 33 percent of adults and teenagers are affected by anxiety disorders in the United States alone. Doctors can have trouble in the diagnosis or may misdiagnose anxiety because all people experience some degree of anxiety in their lives. Anxiety is typical and a normal reaction in certain situations. However, when it becomes the normal primary feeling that is experienced by a person, or when it is affecting his or her life in a negative way, anxiety becomes an issue of mental wellness that can take a physical toll as well. People with high levels of anxiety are prone to feeling like there is a threat even when no threat exists.

When chronic anxiety is present, there is an overflow of stress hormones that are released. The consequences of this can be serious in physical terms. Some of these consequences include the immune system becoming suppressed, the tension of the muscles, and disorders of the digestive system.

There are many other symptoms that can be caused by anxiety. A person who has anxiety may display feelings of unusual tenseness, nervousness, and restlessness. A patient with anxiety may feel that there is impending doom. The person might also feel looming danger or a sense of panic. He or she will always be nervous about what might occur. Physical symptoms of anxiety can occur as well. These can include an acceleration of breathing, an increase in heart rate, sweating, feelings of tiredness, feelings of weakness, or trembling. Much like depression, people who experience anxiety can have difficulties in concentrating. Often times, it can be nearly impossible for the person to even think about anything else besides whatever their current worries or stressors may be. This is evidence of the common combination of anxiety and compulsions.

When a person has an anxiety disorder, there is often a release of an abundance of stress hormones into the bloodstream. These hormones can be the cause of many physical ailments. Not only do these stress hormones suppress the immune system which is a cause of poorer health in general, but they can cause physical symptoms concerning the digestive system, cardiovascular system, and the body's muscles as well. The stress related to anxiety disorders can disrupt your sleep patterns, interfere with your eating habits, and cause you to lose focus or concentration. In addition, stress hormones boost triglycerides, which are fats found in the bloodstream and blood sugar levels as well. Other symptoms that a personal experience as a result of the release of stress hormones are dry mouth, difficulty in swallowing, dizziness, increased heart rate, headaches, fatigue, irritability, tension and achiness in the muscles, nervous energy, nausea, increased rate of breathing, trembling, twitching, and sweating. A person who has chronic anxiety may be more susceptible to developing cardiovascular-related issues, especially at younger ages, even including the risk of a heart attack. Studies have even shown that there is a correlation between anxiety disorders and the development of osteoporosis in women. Osteoporosis is one of the most common and most debilitating metabolic bone disorders in the world. For these reasons listed and many more, it is just as important for physical health as it is for mental wellness to receive adequate treatment when one is suffering from an anxiety disorder.

What Causes Anxiety to be Present in Some People?

It is important to note that a person's anxiety is the result of a combination of factors. Anxiety is not something that is triggered by a single event or as the result of a single factor. Any combination of things can come together to create the perfect conditions for anxiety to be present.

Many factors can play a role in the development of anxiety. Anything from life experiences to personality type to physical health can come into play. Mental health conditions have a tendency to run in families, so having family members who are predisposed to anxiety means that there is a higher likelihood that a person may also develop anxiety. There is a higher chance of a person developing anxiety due to certain characteristics of personality. People with perfectionist tendencies are more likely to have anxiety than those who are not perfectionists. Timid, withdrawn, inhibited individuals are more likely to develop anxiety than their more outgoing counterparts. People who have low self-esteem or who become easily flustered have a higher chance of dealing with anxiety.

Stress is a common predecessor to anxiety. A single instance of stress is not likely to cause a person to develop an anxiety disorder, but ongoing or continuous stress can lead to anxiety. Changing employment or having a high-stress job are often found to be the reason behind anxiety. Family-related events such as pregnancy, childbirth, relationship problems, issues with family, or the death of a loved one can be contributing factors to a diagnosis of anxiety. Any type of trauma or abuse whether verbal, physical, emotional, or sexual can lead a person to develop anxiety. Many stressful events or emotional shock after trauma are also often cited as reasons for the development of anxiety.

Physical conditions such as changes in health and other mental disorders can play a role in the diagnosis of anxiety for a person. Many chronic conditions can contribute to anxiety due to the physical demands that they place on a patient. Diabetes, heart disease, hypertension, and asthma are examples of some of the common conditions that can be co morbid with anxiety. Multiple anxiety disorders can be found at one time in some patients. Other people may be diagnosed with anxiety along with other mental health conditions.

A final noteworthy condition that may predispose people to anxiety is substance abuse. The use of drugs and alcohol can actually contribute to feelings of anxiety. Even if a drug or an alcoholic beverage may seem to help in taking the edge off, as it wears off, the anxious condition is often aggravated.

CHAPTER 1

SIGNS OF TRAUMA

Trauma is the emotional pain that you achieve if you witness failure in any situation. It is the hardline truth seems to be difficult sometimes to endure and if not cured or rectified properly, it could lead you to issues and problems. It is important for you to understand the signs of trauma first then you will be able to manage the trauma in an effective manner. The signs of the trauma are as follows:

1. Anxiety or fear

The anxiety or fear is a sign of trauma through which the person is able to witness pain in his mind and character. When the person is able to achieve anxiety or fear in his character then he should not be able to breathe in a respective manner. The fear of the person is that he will fail in the expectation of the condition and then he will be sad. So, his sadness becomes a source of anxiety for him. Therefore, anxiety is a sign of trauma and the person has to pursue a common mode of affection for the rectification of this sign.

2. Advancements of thoughts

Advancements of thoughts are a terrible sign of trauma for the affected personalities and the persons that have the advancement of thoughts are able to embed themselves in an obscene manner. This advancement of thoughts is a mode of engagement for the people through which the person is able to have laughter on his faith. The advancement of such thoughts comes as a source of brutality for the persons and this advancement enhances when the person is not able to acquire uttermost satisfaction in the case. Advancements can in any reflection in the mind of the person. There is what if skepticism that arises in the mind of the person and he feels terrible while he is asking questions to himself.

3. Being startled by loud noises

There is a startling in the person's mind when he is in a traumatic condition. He thinks as if he has the uttermost satisfaction of the world but actually he is feeling very terrible when he is given a situation to handle. In his internal self, he has lost the situation and he is simply dilly-dallying for no reason. Due to such a menace of situations, a person is able to feel agitated when he even listens to loud noises.

4. Flashback of bad images

There are bad images that come in the mind of a person, who is suffering the worst past. These images resonate a fear mode in the character of the person and he thinks that he has lost the meaning to live. If he has committed an accidental murder, then the image of the body or the dagger or the gun will come to his mind and he will feel ashamed. This flashback tends to demotivate the person from daily routines and he aspires to be nothing in the coming time. These flashbacks ruin a single moment of happiness or dilute euphoric tendencies in the hearts of the people and hence, they become a qualitative source of sadness. Therefore, negative flashbacks are the signs of trauma and sadness for the persons.

5. Physical symptoms

There are also such physical disabilities that come as a result of trauma in a person. There is muscle repairing, bone aching, headaches, sweating and eventful tiredness as well. These symptoms arise from the mental illusion that a person has failed his expectation and he no longer can rise to success. The person is not able to recover from these illnesses and he feels as if it is the end of the world. Physical symptoms no longer give more attention to the people and it is a strong sign of weakness for the persons.

6. Lack of interest in usual activities

When there is trauma in you, you tend to lose interest in every activity that you see around you. You do not want to do sex and you do not seem to have good morale in you when you are in trauma. Sex is just another process for you; you do not seem to have a good sense of relationship with anyone. Therefore, the lack of interest in other activities is a sign of trauma for you.

7. Sleep problems

A person is not able to have a good and relaxing sleeping time when he is in trauma. He feels as if he is in the worst claw of danger and he cannot achieve the best possible way to sleep better. There are bad thoughts that tend to de-motivate the personalities of the persons. While sleeping, a person is able to have a great sense of pleasure when he can sleep. However, a person cannot have this pleasure when he is under tense traumatic conditions.

8. Problems with thinking or concentration

In a traumatic condition, the person is not able to think properly and he feels the audacity to simply run away from the responsibilities. The concentration of the person is very low and he is not able to have a good amount of time with his family or his friends. Thus, there is a token of tension for the persons and he cannot achieve a good amount of relish for himself while he is thinking or concentrating thins.

9. Preoccupation with thinking about trauma

The traumatic effects are so disappointing and distressful that the person becomes preoccupied with the slogan of trauma. He feels that the person is not able to have a good amount of satisfaction for him and there are moments of conflicts that ruin the mundane workability of the persons. The preoccupation is very blistering as it conflicts the person's daily routine in a bad manner. Therefore, trauma is not a manner in which the person can have a good time for himself and the bad preoccupation can lead the person in a degenerate manner.

10. Guilt or self-doubt

Guilt is not able to be transcended in the lives of the persons rather than traumatic effects. It is so dangerous and precarious that the person's ability is tarnished in a bad way. The guilt is able to finish the life of the person and he remains in a self-doubting condition throughout his life. Therefore, in order to be out of trauma, you must not doubt yourself.

CHAPTER 2

PARTS OF THE BRAIN THAT ARE AFFECTED BY THE TRAUMA

Averagely 50% of people will experience traumatic activities at some stage in their lives, but they do not suffer PTSD. The trauma we experience or witness change the functions of the brain at some point more so when someone close to as is struggling to live with their injury. The traumatized brain will coordinate things differently due to the traumatic events they have recorded, the mind is plastic, and it can be changed.

How trauma alters the brain functioning and the parts affected

1. The prefrontal context, this is the thinking center and is located near the behind the forehead it is responsible for the abilities to reason, problem-solving skills, personality, planning and it also makes us aware of ourselves and others. When this part of the brain is functional, we can think clearly and make the right decisions have self-awareness and our environment.
2. The anterior cingulate, it is located just next to the prefrontal cortex but inside the brain. It regulates our emotions and works jointly with the thinking center. When the part is functional, we can manage stressful thoughts that we are experiencing, and also used for

regulating the emotions without being overcome by the feelings and emotions, and this helps us not to participate in the activities that will make us regret later in our lives.

3. And the amygdala, the thin structure found in our brains which act as a fear center, its primary function is to receive information from all our perception organs, and it detects any threat that might be present in our environment and produces fear.

The traumatized brain looks more different compared to the non-traumatized mind

1. The thinking center is under activated
2. The anterior cingulate is under enabled
3. Amygdala is over-activated

Causes of PTSD

Researchers have not concluded the exact cause of PTSD for those who suffer from it; people experience or witness traumatic events, but not all those who experience it suffer PTSD. It is likely a combination of factors that contribute to this, including genetics, personality, life experience, stress, and neurological that provide to other people who have PTSD. The focus to find the cause for PTSD has been its impact on the brain, and it focuses on how the traumatic events have affected the brain functions. Researchers suggest that being overwhelmed by the traumatic events makes the mind not to process any information and not feeling in the right conditions. The traumatic events take control of intruding consciousness, which causes much distress.

There are pre-traumatic psychological factors that may trigger the disorder like low self-esteem, which can worsen the situation. Low self-esteem, which may have been sexually abused, may is much exposed to the PTSD. Post-traumatic reactions from close friends and relatives towards the victims affect them very much, for example, a raped lady is seen as dirty and unclean by the close relatives this causes physical discomfort and flashbacks of the rape events and may influence the persistence of the symptoms. The study of the brain and the mind and its chemical have helped scientist with much information on how the components of the brain and memory contribute to the development of PTSD.

The brain study did focus on the significant two structures of the brain that is: the amygdala and the hippocampus. Amygdala is responsible for fear of how we detect fear in our environment, and it is much hyperactive in those who have PTSD. While the hippocampus is responsible for the formation of memories, there is some placed evidence that those who have PTSD have a loss of volume in the structure and this contributes to the deficits of mind and most of the symptoms of PTSD. Other studies conducted on the neurochemicals that are involved in the cause of PTSD. Hypothalamic pituitary adrenal which is a hormone which is believed to be interrupted within those who have PTSD. It is included in the stress reaction at reasonable rates and its disruption, and its disorder conceptualized as a false alarm.

Hypothalamic pituitary adrenal (HPA) when it is not functional, it re3suts to the damage of hippocampal in those who have PTSD. Medication to this dysfunction reverse to neurochemical dysfunction in those who have PTSD, and they act as agents that switch off the false alarm. It is possible to predict the development of PTSD on early psychological and neurological changes that occur in people exposed to traumatic events.

Risk factors for PTSD

There are numbers of factors that expose people to PTSD, and put people at a higher chance to get PTSD. They include

- Experience or witness a loss at early childhood; this can consist of buses and neglect from families and close relatives or the unknown people.
- Experienced long-lasting trauma, a trauma that does not end, and memories keep on coming to our consciousness.
- Witnessed or underwent severe trauma, like sexual abuse from a close relative or parents during childhood.
- When you view or read a history of mental illness awareness that others are suffering from in their lives.
- You are being in situations that put you at higher risk of

harm like your environmental work situations, for example, those working in the military.

- Experience history of substance or drug abuse like alcohol, this happens when one wants to withdraw from the situation or uses drug abused as coping skills from PTSD.
- History of the mental illness among the family members, genetics where we acquire the genes from our parents. If a parent had PTSD, there is a likely hood that the genes passed to the children.
- When some families or close relatives and friends rely on each other for emotional support, but still they don't get the help from the people they trust.

PTSD Diagnostic and Statistical Manual (DSM)

PTSD wan recognized as a mental illness in 1980, then it was included in the DSM for mental disorders, there was much debate about the disease, but researchers concluded that it is a mental disorder. This was because most of the researchers believed that emotional disturbance after experiencing a traumatic event was regular, but to some people, it results in PTSD and others it did not occur to this PTSD.

PTSD in the DSM-5 Criteria

In DSM-IV and DSM-5, there have been many changes on PTSD, but currently, there are only eight criteria to conclude that someone has PTSD. The first criteria are as follows:

- When one directly experiences the traumatic events. When you interact with the traumatic event straight, for example, sexual abuse or get involved in an accident.
- Witnessing personally the traumatic events how it happened to others, observing how the horrific events happened to a relative, friend or somebody else.
- Getting to know that the traumatic event happened to a close friend, family member, or relatives.
- Re-experiencing traumatic events or too much exposure to traumatic events.

The second criteria for PTSD, which comprises of symptoms involving having repeated of the following:

- Perceptions of our environments
- Images of the traumatic events
- Scary dreams
- Too many illusions and hallucinations, perceiving things that do not exist.
- Flashbacks of the traumatic events that are dissociated.
- Severe psychological distress or anticipating of events to happen.

The third criteria that involve the avoidance of the same stimuli to the traumatic event, avoiding anything that reminds as of the traumatic events.

- Avoiding the thoughts, any feelings, or not talking about the traumatic events we experience.
- Avoiding the factors that might trigger the traumatic memories like avoiding the places, people, or not engaging in any activities that will remind as of the traumatic events we experienced.

The fourth criteria are all about the persistent negative thoughts about traumatic activities.

- One is unable to remember significant events in life, even the once that have been just completed.
- Persistent and overrated negative perceptions about ourselves, others, and our environment.
- Continuously scattered thoughts about the cause of the traumatic event.
- Continuously negative emotional moods.
- Loss of interest to participate in various activities
- Loss of attention from family and friends, feeling detached
- Continuously unable to show positive emotions.

The fifth criteria involve increment of the arousal rates and reactivity

- Displaying irritable behaviors and get angry more often, becomes more irritated very quickly and cannot handle the angry outburst.

- Engages in de3scructive activities as a coping skill.
- Hypervigilance, which increases anxiety.
- Sleep problems have sleep problems not able to sleep properly because of horrific dreams and flashback at night, which are very scary.
- Difficulties in concentrating, attention span is minimal
- Overrated startle response.

And the remaining three criteria

- When the duration of the symptoms is more than 1month, in case the signs are witnessed for more than one month then it can be concluded that the person is suffering from PTSD
- When the disturbances from the memories result in more distress and not able to perform correctly in our daily activities.
- When the disturbance is not as a result of other medical conditions or substance abuse.

Symptoms required to diagnose one who has the PTSD will depend on the criteria listed above.

CHAPTER 3

HOW PAIN, STRESS AND ANXIETY AFFECTS YOUR LIFE

How pain affects your life

At least 100 million Americans, or one in three, live with chronic pain. It's a debilitating condition that affects your ability to work, exercise, focus, relax, do basic household tasks, get a good night's sleep, and fully enjoy life.

Pain can affect your life in numerous ways. If you are a professional and have to go to work, if you experience pain, your work is affected. You will not be able to concentrate on finishing your tasks if something is wrong with you. If you are sick, you have to be absent for treatment or rest. Either way, your work is still affected. If you are a parent, how can you take care of your kids if you are hurt? Pain, is of course a natural stimulus that should not be taken for granted. The more you ignore the pain, the worse your situation may become.

If pain is chronic, it has a detrimental effect on the everyday life of the person. It affects the patient's ability to perform natural functions and responsibilities. Physical activities are limited.

Chronic pain affects you physically and psychologically. It

limits what you can do. It interferes with your ability to work, play with your children or grandchildren; it also diminishes your ability to take care of your own self. When these happen, pain causes you to feel useless and incompetent, making you succumb to a depressed state. People with chronic pain often experience irritability, anger, depression, and difficulty in concentrating. It becomes as debilitating as the pain itself.

It pressures the person while he is trying to hide the pain and forces himself to cover the handicap by a sense of forged well-being to be functional.

Chronic pain is unpredictable. It is sometimes mild and other times, it is unbearable. When a person is in pain, his perception about things is obscured and his responses are slow. This is the stage where a person's personality does not reflect on the outside.

Pain causes sleeplessness and mood swings. Chronic pain leads to painful depressions and helplessness which, in turn leads to suicidal tendencies, anxiety and panic disorders.

If you're in chronic pain, do you notice the effects that it has on your mood and ability to live a normal life? If you have a loved one who suffers from chronic pain, have you noticed changes in them since their pain began?

Chronic pain has become a large-scale public health issue that dramatically worsens quality of life for many people and creates a sizable and growing financial drain on our health care system. The core of the issue is that the medical community does not know how to address the underlying cause of most chronic musculoskeletal pain. Why are drugs and surgery, which are effective roughly 50% of the time, their go-to treatments? The answer that "these are the best solutions we have" is simply not good enough anymore.

People who are in painful situations are always misunderstood. Oftentimes, their real perception and intentions are not reflected on the outside. Their ways of coping with pain is essentially vital to how people view them. Their view of life is also affected. Those who suffer from serious illnesses perceive life as something they have to live to the fullest as their time is already counted and the likes. Some also become hopeless and afraid of the things to come.

The first stop for many pain sufferers is the drugstore, just as the first step for most doctors is to write a prescription for medication. The number of emergency room visits due to overdose of prescription painkillers increased by 34% in just one year between 2016 and 2017. Larger doses of painkillers, often sought by those whose addiction has increased their tolerance for the drug, can cause breathing to slow so much that respiration stops altogether, resulting in a fatal overdose. There are now more overdose deaths involving prescription opioids than there are deaths involving cocaine and heroin combined.

When the structure of the body is damaged beyond the point that rest and improved movement can allow it to repair itself, surgery is typically the best course of treatment. But when function is the issue—as is the case with most people who have chronic musculoskeletal pain—studies consistently indicate that physical rehabilitation is the better choice. It has a higher rate of success, is less expensive, and has far fewer risks than surgery or medication.

To shift out of the surgery-focused trend, some big changes are necessary. Doctors must be educated about the effectiveness of preventive care compared to surgery, and communicate this to their patients. Insurance companies must start covering more types of preventive care. And as a patient, you need to do your part by educating yourself about your condition and getting opinions from multiple doctors. You should also recognize that in many cases there are no magic pills or surgeries that will cure your pain forever. You must put in the work required to take care of yourself on a daily basis so that you can get out of and stay out of pain.

Imaging studies show that regions of the brain involved in making emotional decisions are also involved in chronic pain. To explore this connection, researchers at Northwestern University Medical School and SUNY Upstate Medical University paired chronic back pain patients with healthy control subjects on the Iowa Gambling Task, a card game that measures emotional decision-making abilities. The chronic pain patients performed poorly compared to the control subjects, showing the negative impact chronic pain has on your ability to make decisions.

Another major challenge is that people suffering from chronic pain tend to feel like they have no understanding or control over their pain. Despite all that modern medicine knows about the human body, the medical community still understands relatively little about pain—so much so that 85% of lower back pain sufferers receive no definitive diagnosis.

How Stress and Anxiety Affects Your body and Life

There can be situations when you just cannot act like before you used to because now anxiety has taken a grip of you. It is the feeling of being afraid of the unknown. On a broader sense, anxiety comes in different forms sometimes feeling worried, apprehensive, being nervous or plainly everything going out of control. Severe forms of anxiety can be extremely devastating and can have a great impact on your life and health.

Fear and panic are natural human emotions. Everyone has felt anxious for one reason or another. It is the feeling of worry, apprehension or panic in response to certain situations which is usually unsafe or uncomfortable.

Anxiety is a basic human emotion. Generally speaking, it is healthy and manageable to a certain degree. Because everyone experiences anxiety, it can be challenging to recognize and accept anxiety as a problem, however if you just ignore the symptoms of anxiety, you miss the chance to understand your life and yourself better. If you try to understand what your anxiety is telling you, you will have a better chance of overcoming the problem. In effect, you get to enjoy a better quality of life.

Is your anxiety helping you or has it become excessive and detrimental? We'll now try to learn more about anxiety and what you can do to help control the problem.

There are several 'listed' disorders that are all classified as 'anxiety.' Depending on the duration of the anxiety and its severity, it can actually lead to physical symptoms. When it manifests physically, it can cause the person to feel worn out, rundown, fatigued, it can cause pain in muscles and joints, it can lead to an increased risk of getting sick, and it can even increase the risk of heart attack, stroke, and a number of other health emergencies.

There are probably plenty of things that you have gone through in your life that caused you some level of worry. Maybe you had a test in high school that worried you. Even if you studied and felt confident that you knew the material, you might have worried about that test.

Maybe it kept you from getting a good night's sleep right before that test. Would that be considered anxiety?

It all depends. Since it interfered with your ability to sleep, some people could have been diagnosed as having mild anxiety. But most likely once the test was over you were able to get back to your normal routine and didn't worry about it anymore, and that wouldn't be classified as anxiety. More like stress.

We all experience stress throughout our life. It's quite natural and normal, but when you begin to worry excessively about certain things, especially things that you cannot control, then it becomes a problem.

As you deal with stress on a regular basis, whether it's because of financial pressures, schooling, relationship problems, worries about your job or finding work, or anything else, it can develop into anxiety over time.

What usually happens is that the worry starts to consume your thoughts. You begin thinking about the challenges you're facing on a regular basis. You could be thinking about the rent that's late while driving home from work knowing you can't possibly pay it right now.

You could be worried about the company you work for downsizing. You might be concerned about your adult child's well-being because he's out partying every night, doesn't seem to be taking any responsibility for his life, is getting himself into debt, and nothing you say or do –aside from paying those bills for him-is making a difference.

When you try to fall asleep at night, when the TV is off and everything is quiet, you can't shut the worry and stress off. You keep turning those fears over and over in your mind.

At some point in the middle of the night you might finally drift off to sleep but the alarm blares just two or three hours later. Now you're tired and have the deal with another day like that. Multiply that night after night and the anxiety will continue to build even more because now you're trying to focus at work, impress the boss, or getting impatient with people around you. You might snap at somebody then feel bad about it right away, and that's going to make things worse in your mind. Eventually you may feel tightness in your chest, shortness of breath at times, and have a difficult time getting anything done.

Over time you might withdraw from some of the activities you used to enjoy because you're spending all of your time worrying about everything, even though you're not actually able to do anything about them.

In time, you're living a completely different life with little to enjoy. That can lead to depression and a general state of worry about many other things, even those things that weren't a major concern for you in the past.

CHAPTER 4

HOW TO DEAL WITH TRAUMA

The following are some of the mechanisms through which traumas can be dealt with properly.

1. Safety first

Safety is the most crucial factor when it comes to deal with trauma. If you are a person that is dealing with trauma be sure that you are in a safe position with your families. By safety, it is argued that the person is able to have an emotional satisfaction for himself and he can get a good intake of help and productivity for others. The safety factor needs to be adopted so that the person is not able to have a strong safe environment for himself. Therefore, the safety first assertion is a method that can be used to have a prosperous factor for himself. So, safety needs to be strengthened in order to make the traumatic person feel great.

2. Talking with someone you trust

While you are in a trauma, you need to talk with someone, who could give you more input about your character. You have to be more lenient with others while you are facing a traumatic condition. The talking factor will help to reduce all your engines and tensions and will make you feel more comfortable and compatible with any worst situation you encounter.

3. Knowing that your feeling is very normal for someone

The feeling for someone will be very normal for you then you have to leave him/her for good reasons. You must understand that you need to love others for a good reason but be careful so that you can be more and more insightful in this regard. Always remember that you have a strong potential deeply hidden in you and you need to extract it by all means necessary.

4. Accepting the belief

This paragraph advocates that you have to understand the present scenario of yourself and try yourself to get rid of all the quagmires that are haunting you. You have to be pertinent in your manner and must accept the strength so that you may understand the presence of the scintillating present in front of you. You have to believe that the acceptance will bring upon a greater version of strength and sustenance for yourself.

5. You have to spend time doing relaxing things

The relaxation is important for you so that you may understand the primaries of life in a better manner. You can go for a walk, you may look upon substantial things in your daily routine like listening to music, baking food for others and even talking things in a perpetual manner. The relaxation of yourself is highly crucial for you to understand the primaries of life and you may look upon great measures of life in a pertinent manner. This is the moment of relaxation for you and you may have a great zeal for yourself if you do relaxing things in life.

6. Confronting the situations in an effective and disciplined manner

You have to confront the situations in front of you that were haunting and horrific for you in the past. The situations might be very degenerate and deplorable for you if you do not have the ability to decipher the wrong times and understand that bad times do not last for long. Bad times teach you to be strong and sustainable and if you have guts in yourself then you will rise in these conundrums by hook or by crook. Therefore, the confrontation with the past is a mode that can be helpful for you to attain more salvation and solace for you by all means necessary.

7. Do not use drugs and alcohols to cope up with

Some nihilists of life and process believe that drugs can give you a great sense of affection so that you may forget the pawns of life and become more estranged from responsibilities. The drugs might have a temporary effect on your body and it may momentarily affect the conditions of your mind but in the true sense, it is very harmful and dangerous for the cognition and metabolism for the body. It is important for you that you understand that drugs are the extractors of happiness and they induce a conflicting mode of competitiveness among you and make you fall in despair and distrust. Therefore, in order to curb the mechanism of trauma, please refrain from the use of drugs.

8. Education to the patients

The doctor is also an educationalist, who must be able to give an exciting speech or an educating spree of messages to the personalities that can be in the condition of the trauma and there needs to be more and more insightful to the persons, who want the ideas of a better life and this above all must be the underlines message by the doctor to the people, who are prone to traumas. This message or mental conciliation will help the doctors and the patients to learn the happiness of life and within time, they would be able to give more and more insight into the matter.

So, these are some of the tactics and methods that can be used to give patients the moments of happiness and adaptability for the person. These could be the illustrations for the people that are traumatic and with the passage of time; they will be able to understand the mindsets of the public.

CHAPTER 5

COMPLEX PTSD BEHAVIOR AND HOW TO CONTROL IT

Complex PTSD: Beyond Trauma.

Since childhood, many of us have heard stories and watched movies about the mental disorders suffered by almost all of World War II survivors, known as Post-traumatic Stress Disorder. However, anyone can suffer from this disease, from children to the elderly.

Complex Post-traumatic Stress Disorder (complex PTSD) involves the presence of PTSD with added problems of self-regulation in the person, where they do not control their actions and become someone very different. It usually occurs in people who have experienced multiple traumatic events, a prolonged trauma or an especially severe trauma (usually related to interpersonal victimization).

One of many examples of complex PTSD, according to Luxenberg et al. (2001), would be a woman who as a child never received the necessary care and attention, with an alcoholic stepfather who raped her on many occasions, and saw her stepfather rape her mother (vicarious victimization).

Behavior behind complex PTSD

The main alterations that differentiate complex PTSD from PTSD lie in a person's inability to self-regulate. This involves changes in several mental aspects, but to regulate the symptoms we suffer, our behavior must change.
Some of the changes observed are:

1) Self-harm.

Some people look for any way to alleviate their pain and emotional suffering, and sometimes they get it through self-harm. Most of these attitudes develop during trauma, when perhaps the experience is so negative that they want to take their own lives.

2) People-pleasers

In a desperate attempt to avoid any uncomfortable or negative situation that may affect their fragile emotional state, some people with complex PTSD become almost servants, seeking to please every act and submit to activities unpleasant for themselves, trying to live also through the pleasure of others.

3) Isolation

The inability to maintain interpersonal relationships due to chronic distrust and living angry or full of hostility, leads some people to isolate themselves. When this is reversed, it often symbolizes a strong point in the recovery process.

4) Addictions

Self-medication is not unique to complex PTSD to get into alcohol or drugs, many people create addictions to these substances because of other issues. However, in this case, it is part of the defense mechanisms created by the individual to deal with or try to forget their trauma.

5) Temperament

Many people with Complex PTSD can become aggressive, when criticized they cannot tolerate any opinion or will react in a volatile manner to the smallest criticism. These are not common reactions in them; rather they differ from their original personality and trigger emotional instability, dragging them into loneliness.

How to maintain control over yourself

There are many measures that can help you control symptoms and your reaction to situations, among them:

- Become familiar with your illness: look for information about complex PTSD and its symptoms, the more you know about your condition, the more confident you will feel.

- Look for your "safe person" a trusted person who will listen to you and help you on this journey.
- Self-help groups: As you already know, there are many PTSD and Complez PTSD groups. If you don´t already have one, look for one, attend, and share your experience. They will help you to manage your anger and lessen the impact of your trauma on you. Remember, sharing your feelings is the best way to free yourself.
- Avoid drug or alcohol use: remember that drugs and alcohol will never help long-term and in moments of difficulty they are extra dangerous. Don't sabotage yourself.
- Get professional help: it will improve your acceptance of yourself and give you tools to deal with your disorder. This is essential for your recovery.
- Talk to your family or to close friends if possible, they can play a key role in your recovery. While they should give you space, they should also give you support.
- Be patient: Change will not happen overnight. Do not worry or anguish yourself, you will get better and your pain will subside, if you persevere. Complex PTSD is like everything in life, it takes time and patience to master it.

CHAPTER 6

COGNITIVE BEHAVIORAL THERAPY TOOLS FOR ANXIETY

There are many pills that you can take for anxiety. Unfortunately, these are just temporarily reliefs that won't fix the root problem.

There's a chance that by this point, you are already feeling a little bit better. Sometimes, all it takes is sharing and confronting your feelings for you to have a better sense of yourself and the things that trigger you. Telling just one person about a trauma, a secret, or something that you fear can make you feel better. Having to keep that all in yourself can cause a lot of strain. That's added responsibility that you might not always have the mental capacity for.

It all starts with identifying your root causes. Is it body image issues from society or your parents? Did you have abusive family members that hurt you physically and mentally? Perhaps it was a great trauma that has led to depression and anxiety in your adult life.

Make sure that you are taking notes on what those are. If something pops into your head, jot it down so you can look back at it later. Remember that you aren't going to be able to unravel it all right away. At first, you might just be able to look back at your life and see the loss of a parent as the root cause for some issues. Once you explore that, you will discover other small instances that experience affected and how that has resulted in the way that you think today.

After you have identified the root cause, you can start to see how it has manifested itself into your life. Do you experience obsessive-compulsive disorder after parental abandonment? Do you have social anxiety because of your body image issues? When we look at the 'what' of our mental illness, we can look at the 'why', and vice versa. Sometimes, you might first notice your habits before the cause, or maybe you already know the cause and can now use that to explain your behavior now. Either way, it is important to make sure that you are aware of this so you can come up with specific cognitive behavioral therapy tools to overcome that.

Now, it is time to start to see what we can do to turn these thoughts and feelings around. Instead of finding a quick fix, we have to look at long-term solutions to help us overcome fear and anxiety. These are all methods that aren't going to solve all your problems right away. They are things that you need to practice, but with time, they become easier. It took a while to develop the automatic thoughts you have now, so you can't expect that they'll stop after reading this book. After a while, however, you will find that they come naturally to you.

Mindfulness

Mindfulness is going to be one of the most helpful tools for all forms of mental illness. Whether you are anxious all the time, or just experience social anxiety in situations with other people around, you can benefit from mindfulness. It can be helpful for those that have constant depressive thoughts as well.

It can be easy to run away with your thoughts when you are feeling stressed and overwhelmed. You might escape to a place in your mind, real or not, where you don't have to think about the present. It might be a fantasy of a life that's better than the one you are living, or perhaps you often reminisce on times that were better than now.

Mindfulness is the attempt to ground you and keep you in reality, rather than lost in your anxious and stressful thoughts. When you think of one anxious thing, it can easily lead to many other worries. For example, you might think, "Oh no, I have to pay the cable bill because it is already late." Then you might start thinking of all the other bills stacking up, not to mention the debt that's increasing in interest. Then you start to think about how you aren't making enough money at your current job, or that you should have gone to school for a different subject, or you shouldn't have broken up with that guy who's now a doctor. One thought about a late cable bill can lead to an existential crisis if you don't stop anxiety right in its tracks. Mindfulness will help you through this. Instead of ruminating on what could have, would have, or should have been, you instead focus on the now, which is really what is most important.

It is something that needs to be practiced. You might only be able to be comfortably mindful for a few seconds at a time before your thoughts go straight back to something else. When you find that you are losing yourself in your own thoughts, you have to make sure that you redirect. Back to the example of the cable bill, you might notice your anxiety rising when you think of the other bills stacking up. That is when you would stop your thoughts and instead use a mindful tactic to bring you back to the present and instead focus on the cable bill.

Then, you might find that your mind is wandering again, and before you know it, you are thinking about that wealthy guy and what could have been. You have not failed, but you just need to redirect again, either using a new mindful technique or just practicing the other one again. Don't punish yourself for drifting back into those thoughts.

Picture yourself driving down a highway. The present is the road in front of you, the past the grass to the right, and the future the other road on the left. If you drift too far right or left, then you'll get lost and off track. Mindfulness is what's going to keep you moving forward in the right direction. At first, you are going to be driving down the road very wobbly. Every time you feel yourself drift off to the right or the left, redirect and focus back on going straight. Eventually, you'll find it very easy to avoid drifting at all.

Mindfulness should be practiced whenever you find that you

are experiencing symptoms of anxiety. You should practice mindfulness even when you aren't in a negative mindset. Maybe you are just bored or restless, which are also forms of anxiety. We don't always view being bored as a bad thing, and many people feel lucky if they get the chance to have nothing to occupy their time. If you are bored for too long, however, you might find your thoughts drifting somewhere dangerous, so practice mindfulness even if you don't feel like you are that obviously anxious.

The below three sections are different forms of mindfulness that you should practice as often as possible. Even if you aren't feeling totally anxious, you can still use these to help prevent future moments of anxiety. No harm will come from mindfulness. These aren't the only methods of mindfulness either.

Some activities would be considered mindful, such as playing a game or reading a book. Anything that keeps your mind on the present is going to be mindful. We might not always have the time to play a game or read a book to pull us out of our thoughts, however, so it is important to remember to use these tools for when you are feeling anxious.

Five Senses

Your five senses are your ability to see, smell, taste, hear, and touch. When being mindful, a good form is to go through each of these senses to feel better. This activity starts by sitting somewhere comfortably, preferably with your feet flat on the floor. When you are in a comfortable place, it is easier for your mind to focus on what it needs to. You might be feeling anxious at work, waiting at the doctor's office, or just in your own home. No matter where you are, you can go through this process to help ground you and keep you in the moment, avoiding anxious and depressive automatic thoughts.

First is your sight. Find five things that you can see. This is just simply anything that is in your range of eyesight. It might be the rug that your feet are on or the building you see out the window. Perhaps it is the table with things sitting on them and all the stuff that's on top. Whatever your five items are, it doesn't matter. The only thing you have to do is identify them.

Next, identify four things that you can smell. Don't actually get up from where you are sitting to smell them. Just try to pick them out. Maybe it is the coffee sitting on the counter or a manhole you see walking down the street. Perhaps you imagine smelling the cat, or the candy sitting in the dish on the table.

Look for three things to touch. These are easily identifiable things. It might include the couch you are sitting on, your own hair, or your pants. Maybe it is just something across the room, like a salt lamp, or a soft scarf hanging on the coat rack. You don't have to touch these things either. Just think about what three things you could touch.

Find two things you could hear. This could include the birds chirping outside or the music softly playing on the elevator. Perhaps it is the tapping of someone else's foot or the sound of nails scraping on a table. Whatever these are, pick them out.

Pick out one thing that you can taste. This isn't something that has to be edible either. Maybe it is the taste of the water from a fountain in front of you or a sandwich someone else is eating. No matter what it is, everything has a flavor, edible or not, and your goal is to just identify that taste.

You don't actually have to do these activities. You don't have to taste something or smell something. But identifying it as something that you could use that for can be enough to pull you back into the moment. You don't have to go in that order either. Instead, you can try finding five things to touch, four things to hear, three things to taste, two things to smell, and one thing to see. Just remember your five senses and a descending amount.

If you don't have one of these senses, such as the ability to hear, see, or taste, then simply replace that with another sense. Either way, the goal is to give you something you can identify in the moment so that you are pulled away from the anxious thoughts in the first place.

Finding Colors

Another activity for mindfulness is to search for one specific color. When you are feeling anxious, think of one color. It shouldn't be something specific at first, just simply pick something like blue, black, gray, white, or yellow.

Look around the room and pick out everything that is that color. This doesn't have to be done in any specific order. Simply look for things that are red, or green, or any other simple color. Again, if you don't have this ability and are color blind, try using a different "rule." Maybe you find only things that are made of metal, or you pick out all the things made of wood.

Identify what might be a close sister of that color. After picking out all the green stuff, look at that specifically and think about what's lime green, what's forest green, and everything in between.

Before you know it, your mind is on something completely different than what was making you anxious. There are no rules to this either. If you miss an item, nothing bad will happen. The goal is to get your brain to stop thinking about what's causing anxiety and instead look directly toward what's around you at the current moment.

If it isn't working at first, try repeating with a different color. Do this after you do the five senses, or vice versa. Come up with your own games too, like identifying all the things that make white noise, or the things that you can smell that are made of wood. The only thing you have to make sure you are doing is that you are focusing on the now and not on the past or future.

Muscle Relaxation

When we're anxious, it can be hard to realize just how much we might be using our muscles. Your back, jaw, neck, shoulders, and other parts of your body that are responsible for support can be sore often if you don't properly manage your anxiety. There are even some people that believe certain pains are associated with certain issues, such as lower back and hip pain being caused by money issues. This isn't proven by science, but it is interesting to think about just how much pain we might be feeling simply because of our anxiety.

Tensing and releasing your muscles is a good form of mindfulness that keeps you focused on the now, and that will help your body feel better afterward too. It involves identifying your muscles and tensing them for three to five seconds, and then holding for one to two seconds in between, focusing on deep breathing the entire time. Don't push yourself if it is too straining, and skip over any muscles that might be sore or parts of your body with too much nerve damage. The point isn't to strain yourself, but to focus instead on how tense you are and how to relieve that tension.

Start with your head. Clench your jaw for a few seconds and then release. Raise your ears and hold them tight or tilt your neck to each side for a few seconds. Move down to your shoulders, raising them up as high as possible and then dropping them as much as you can. Just when you think you have relaxed your shoulders, relax them even more.

Now, move onto your chest and arms. Hold them tight for a few seconds, releasing for a few afterward. The entire time, make sure that you are fully breathing in and out so that you don't lose your breath. Then, go to your stomach, legs, feet, and repeat if you need to. It is not supposed to be a workout, but just a way for you to become aware of how tense you might be. Our muscles can become very sore if we don't properly hold them right.

Between each of these muscle tightening moments, make sure to take a deep breath in and let it out slowly. Count your breathing and count how long you are holding. Consistency will help regulate your heart and lungs so that those too help with overall anxiety reduction.

This is why exercising can be so relaxing for many people. It gets your mind focused on something else and also keeps the blood pumping. Remember that exercise is healthy and important, but it can also be a source of anxiety. Don't put pressure on yourself to be physical right away, especially if that's one of your triggers. The gym can be a scary place, and even walking down the street can cause people to panic, so while it is important to keep your body moving to avoid anxious symptoms, don't make yourself feel bad that you aren't in a place where you can do this.

CHAPTER 7

HOW TO USE TAPPING TO REDUCE PTSD

Trauma and Safety

Trauma and safety in the brain.

A Biological and Emotional Perspective

If the information seems sad, the amygdala puts a sad stamp on it, categorizing it as sad. If anger seems like the dominant emotion in the event, the amygdala will categorize it as angry. Generally, memories then move on to the hippocampus, the hard drive of the brain where they're stored in memory. However, with trauma, the memories don't necessarily move into the hippocampus. They hang out by the amygdala. This is what allows them to get retriggered when additional sensory information is processed by the thalamus. That's when what you may be seeing, hearing, or touching remind you of the trauma. The trauma hasn't been put in storage. It's hanging out by the amygdala where it's easily accessible, and that's what allows us to be retriggered. We don't feel safe because of our ability to get so easily retriggered. It's very hard for us to relax because we're on edge as a result of these unprocessed memories. Tapping helps us clear the charge, allowing the memory to move into storage so the nervous system can relax and we feel safer.

An Energetic Perspective

From an Eastern medicine perspective and the tapping perspective, all disease—physical, mental, emotional, or spiritual—is caused by a block in the flow of energy through the body. Energy flows through via meridian lines, which are like electrical lines that bring the energy to all the different parts of the body (Solomon, 2007). That's what allows us to sustain our health and well-being. When that energy gets disrupted, that's what causes illness. That's what trauma is—the stuck energy. This is what causes us to feel unsafe. With tapping, we are getting this energy unstuck and restoring its flow.

We can see from both the biological brain and energetic perspectives that stuck energy is what's keeping us feeling unsafe and causing us to have difficulty relaxing.

Trauma in the Chakras

The chakra system.

Trauma affects the root chakra. We all have seven chakras, which are energy centers in the body that govern different life issues. The root chakra governs safety and security (Judith & Jenner, 2016). When trauma occurs, our sense of safety and security is disrupted. The root chakra is also the closest to the earth. When our root chakra is open and activated, it allows us to ground and feel connected to the earth. When we're ungrounded, we start to feel anxiety because we're no longer tethered and anchored to the earth properly. The root chakra and our ability to be grounded is part of what helps us to be present in our lives. When trauma happens, often we feel unsafe being present in the here and now. There's a subconscious fear that what happened may happen again. Perhaps we don't like being here because we have to feel the discomfort of the trauma stored in the body, so we want to leave. We leave the present moment and become depressed—stuck in the past or worried about the future.

Trauma and Addiction

We use addiction to cover over the pain and discomfort of being present. Whether the addiction is drugs, alcohol, sex, or television, it helps us avoid having to deal with the pain and discomfort of being here now.

The Most Important Reason to Create Safety: The Window of Tolerance

window of tolerance.

The window of tolerance is the most important reason for safety when we're doing trauma work (Siegel, 2012). The middle box is also called the window of tolerance; this is what we're able to tolerate. If we're able to tolerate what it is that we're experiencing, we stay in the window of tolerance.

If we start getting agitated and anxious, we get what's called **hyperarousal**. This is where we become emotionally reactive and snap at people. This is also where we start to feel anger, rage, and become hypervigilant, constantly on guard for danger.

We can also go in the other direction—toward the bottom—which is **hypoarousal**. You can think of this as underarousal where we numb out, freeze, or shut down to cope with the situation.

We want to be able to maintain a sense of safety while we're doing trauma work by staying in this window of tolerance. Otherwise, if we venture into hypoarousal or hyperarousal, we have to stop doing any healing. If that happens, we're unable to be lucid and present enough to do meaningful work and experience the healing benefits. Safety is super important to help us stay in that window of tolerance.

How to Create Safety: Resourcing

Resourcing is exactly what it sounds like. It's where we give the system what it needs to have its needs met and to relax (Spiers, 2001). With trauma, the system is often underresourced. Meaning, the way that we experience this is feeling like we don't have the tools to cope. We feel unsafe, but we don't know what to do to create safety. It's like if I ask you to make a peanut butter and jelly sandwich, but you don't know where the bread or the peanut butter or the jelly is, and you don't know what a knife is.

Many Different Ways to Resource Yourself

1. Having a cup of tea
2. Taking a bath
3. Getting enough sleep
4. Taking breaks
5. Eating healthy and staying hydrated
6. Making sure food, water, and bathroom access are available
7. Creating connection with another person
8. Practicing meditation and guided meditation

These are some different ways to resource yourself (Spiers, 2001). Notice that there are two main themes here. Having a cup of tea and taking a bath and meditation all help to relax the system. Getting enough sleep, eating healthy, and making sure that food, water, shelter, and bathroom access are available all have to do with making sure that our basic needs are met. When those basic needs are met, our system innately feels safer. As a result, we can do more in our lives, and we can do healing work as well.

Guided Meditation

The main method that I like for resourcing is guided meditation. It's something you can do when you have your phone with you or if you have access to a laptop. It's something you could do while you're sitting and you have a few minutes at home, on a bus, or in a public setting. All you need are headphones. Guided meditation is where someone uses his or her voice to guide you through a process with a specific intention, usually by visualizing certain things (Call, 2010). Guided meditation can be used to relax, to meet your spirit guide or higher self, or to create safety. I like guided meditation for resourcing because it's very intentional. We are going into it with the intention of creating safety, and it gives us a designated activity to do that on a daily basis and during trauma work. It's something we can incorporate directly into the healing work, compared to something like drawing a bath where we have to run the water and wait a little while. For tea, we have to have the tea, a cup, and access to hot water. As long as we have a phone or a laptop, we can do a guided meditation at any time while we're working through trauma.

CHAPTER 8

THE DISTRACTOR DISPUTING

Distract, and Dispute method is a method used to overcome the beliefs from the ABCs. It is a more natural way to overcome the way we react towards the things or situations thrown our way. Someone who can control their emotions and how they hold any challenges is an optimistic person. They try to see the good even when the situation does not allow. A pessimistic person, on the other hand, holds very negative beliefs.

What determines if you are optimistic or pessimistic is the belief you hold after a situation. One is supposed to learn how to handle ABCs positively.

Distracting

Before the negativity overwhelms you, it is important to distract yourself. When you face a difficult situation and feel that your mind is about to go the negative way of thinking, find a distraction by doing something else. One can find something that distracts them every time they need the distraction. Like when the negatives begin to come your way, you can pinch yourself as a reminder that you are supposed to let go of those thoughts.

Disputation

The most permanent way to deal with negative thoughts is by disputing them. Dispute the thoughts by dealing with the negativities head-on instead of interrupting them. Interrupting is short-lived as it means temporarily avoiding thinking about the situation. You may succeed interrupting several times, but until you have dealt with the issue by disputing, it will keep recurring.

When you have dealt with the activities that make your beliefs, then seen the consequences and disputed the beliefs, the next stage that comes is the new effects. Someone now has better consequences because they already disputed the beliefs. The ABC model is very accommodating because other than your change towards how you react in different circumstances, everything else is constant. You don't have to change anything else, including your environment.

Behavioral Exercises

These are exercises used to get samples of someone to determine their real conduct so that certain of his skills can be tested. Behavioral exercises usually are used for assessing for the recruitment process. The following are some of the types of behavioral exercises that are sometimes used together with someone's own psychological computation.

Group exercises – this is a determined personal ability to interact with others how you engage with your group mates when trying to solve an issue together. The group work is credited to an individual score for all the members to find how effective they are in a group setting.

Presentation exercise – how one carries themselves, especially considering that all the attention is on them. Some may find it extremely difficult to be in front of people.

Role plays – A person in a group is given a role to play out a specific role. How one plays in this role is crucial because it means they can handle the pressure.

360 surveys – this will depend on how the members of the group will credit him. What do the others think are their strengths and weaknesses?

Anxiety and trauma

how they performed in their previous works, the roles they played and how they performed in their respective past roles.

Performance at the assessment center exercise – a candidate, in this case, is sent to an office where the assessors give him tasks to do, and they have to do precisely what they are told. They may be given any work from any field and how they can handle it will determine the final results for the score of that day.

Inbox exercise – this is used to determine how well a person can take care of items belonging to the group in a short time of period.

Interviews – A candidate is given the task of talking about a real-life situation where they had to deal with a certain task to show their suitability. They are supposed to come up with examples of instances about a particular topic where they were put under pressure to prove their skills.

Metacognitive Techniques

Metacognitive Therapy is a theory that claims that people have beliefs about their ways of thinking, and usually the beliefs are incorrect. People sometimes have positive beliefs regarding worry. Most people argue that worrying protects them. They feel that with worry, it keeps them alert of situations they would have foreseen had they been unworried. There are also negative beliefs regarding worry. One may feel that no matter how much they worry, they may not be able to do anything about it. People also sometimes think that worry will sink them into depression.

The problem with the negative thoughts is that even if we had control over the worry, we are unlikely to do anything about it because we have the belief that we cannot do anything about it. This is where metacognitive therapy comes in. It counters these beliefs "meta" beliefs. Metacognitive therapy claims that, if we could get rid of the worries, to begin with, do away with the perception that there is no way we cannot get rid of worrying it gets easier to deal with the worries head-on.

Metacognitive therapy tops are an addition of cognitive-behavioral therapy. While cognitive deals with our thoughts, Metacognitive deals with the thoughts of our thoughts. In cognitive-behavioral therapy, we ask ourselves about what will happen if we take some risks, find out the possibilities of bad things happening as well as the right things and what would be the results. In metacognitive, we question the process. We ask ourselves why we should worry about it while we may not be helpful at all.

Metacognition helps in:

It helps people comprehend and be in power to control their cognitive performance.

People are given authority and charge over their learning. This is by exposing to them their best learning method, the progress of their learning, strategies that will improve their learning and ways of using the strategy to achieve the best results possible.

Boosts the self-confidence of a learner because metacognitive skills help them with the skills to think critically and also make the best decisions

A person can use metacognitive skills even outside of school. It is applicable in the outside world and not just for students.

Metacognitive therapy is for every age group. The young and the old can all apply the skills in their day to day activities. It helps all age groups be self-reflectors and hard thinkers

It helps in the reduction of stress as it eliminates all the self-doubts and also gives ways to avoid worries.

Metacognition Has Two Processes That Help Learners Remember It.

- Knowledge of cognition- has three factors; awareness of factors that influence individual performances, Identifying different strategies to help deal with learning, Identifying the best solution in a learning situation.
- Regulation of cognition – this includes having the right goals set and planning strategically, observing and controlling learning, self-evaluation to check on the overall personal performance.

Metacognitive Requires Three Common Strategies Which Include:

- Arranging and planning
- Centering
- Evaluating

1. Arrangement And Planning

This has five techniques that help to learn, study and practice.

Learning about learning – here, you find out your strengths and weaknesses when learning.

It also involves planning a task of what exactly you want to do.

Make the proper time arrangements to cater for your targeted goals and tasks.

Knowing what the purpose of your task is, is equally very important because you will be able to execute them in the best way possible.

2. Centering

This requires paying maximum attention to everything you are being taught. You also make sure to listen carefully at everything being communicated to you, whether formally or informally. When you pay attention, it means you grasp information subconsciously that you may miss if you do not pay attention. How much you learn depends on how much attention you paid when you were being taught. When you center, you can have a subconscious overview of a particular topic.

3. The self-evaluation, also known as self-monitoring.

You sit back and think of all the progress you have made. You may think you are making progress when you are not and evaluating will give you the feedback of if you are. During self-evaluation, you may discover things like your strengths and weakness in different topics so that you don't proceed as if you know, while you don't understand anything or haven't learned anything.

Metacognitive skills are essential in students as it helps them improve their way of thinking so that they can comfortably learn on their own and improve their life and school experiences. It's important for young people to be able to solve issues, be sharp thinkers, be efficient communicators, and be able to relate with their peers and everyone properly.

Being metacognitive means, holding back and think before making rushed decisions. You make sure to observe you're possible actions and see how you can react differently. You first begin by identifying the problem, find out the strategy to deal with the problem because every problem demands a different reaction, the progress you have made in trying to find a solution for your problem, how you can improve in a situation the next time it happens. With these questions, you can engage your brain in a more profound, broad way of understanding situations so that you make responsible decisions.

Strategies Of Teaching Students To Use Metacognition

- Defining the term let them explain how they understand metacognition and how they think they can apply it in their real life.
- 2.students should talk about the benefits they believe

metacognition will impact in their life. This could be understood in writing where an analysis of a passage is well done to make sure the information is well communicated.

- Help the students apply metacognition even as they interact with their peers. They may be paired in groups and asked to come up with benefits of how metacognition in a group.
- The students can discuss how metacognition can be used in the outside world as well as inside the school.
- Use problems to help students know how if dealt with a similar situation how they can deal with it.

Metacognition Skills That One May Apply In Life.

Metacognition skills are essential for a learner because it produces successful learners if they adhere to them.

- One should be able to understand their limits as learners. This involves knowing how much your memory can accommodate when dealing with a particular task and getting away for external help.
- Self-evaluating the method you use to learn taking notes of all its effectiveness and then changing where there needs to be changed so that the strategy works out well.
- Taking notes of everything you need and then noting where you didn't understand. Recording what you

understood will help you not to forget while what you didn't realize you can work on later.

- Ignoring the information that is not important to you so that you can concentrate on what is useful to you.
- Put what you know into practice so that you don't end up forgetting what you already knew.
- Regularly taking tests to see how far you have progressed.

Since metacognitive involves 'learning how to learn' there are a few ways to achieve this:

- Asking questions is essential for learners to reflect on what they have learned and how well their strategies are working for them. In a group set up, ask the students to think about the role they would play when solving conflicts in the team.
- It is essential to insist that the students do a self-reflection on the progress they had made before they learned about metacognitive and after they got exposed to it. Self-analyzing on personal progress will allow self-criticism and therefore be a great expanding process to learn.
- Encouraging learners to ask questions is very important. They should generate their questions and answer to the best of their knowledge as this will also help in knowing and understanding the depth of the

knowledge they have.

- Teach relevant metacognitive strategies to the class as part of the regular learning.
- Challenge your learners to come up with their metacognitive strategies as a way of promoting independent learning.
- Encourage the practice of metacognitive strategies in groups so that they sit and discuss them in groups. This will help them learn from one another and also be able to solve problems as one.
- Providing mentors is very important because students tend to relate more to topics when they are dealing with their peers. The mentors can talk about the metacognitive strategies that worked for them and how they handled them and how it worked for them. This might inspire someone in the class or create a broader understanding than before they met the mentors.
- Letting learners know the importance of thinking their thoughts aloud and also reporting the thoughts they encountered while handling a difficult issue. When someone speaks aloud their thoughts, they can receive help in places they may have been struggling with. You will also get an opinion from others which perfect feedback to know how far you real have come from.
- Self-explaining for learners may help improve the

understanding of a rather tricky topic. It may be done in writing or in speaking as long as someone can clearly understand the situation after they have expressed themselves.

- It is okay for learners to know that making mistakes is still okay, and no one can be crucified for mistakes. Making mistakes is part of the learning process, and learners can correct them and move forward progressively.

In simple terms, what happens in a metacognitive strategy can be summarized as below.

1. Planning and organizing – what a planner should do is to strategically set their goals, plan the strategy of the task, find ways in which you intend to accomplish your task by finding the best strategies, make a preview. When all this accomplished, the planning and organizing part has been well accomplished, and it is time to go to the next step.
2. Observe and identify the problems – while working on a task, it's essential to keep checking the progress of the said task, check your understanding on the topic to see how much you have understood, try to see if you are sensible in your job because you may end up with a task that does not make any sense.
3. Evaluating- after you are done with a task, look back at how much you have achieved on the job, look back at

how best you have utilized the learned strategies, identify how applicable the strategy you have used are, look at different styles you could use the next time you undertake a similar or separate task. Learning from the mistakes, you think you have made on the job so that the next time you take a task, you don't repeat the mistakes.

4. Managing your learning – identify your style. People learn differently; what works for someone else might not work for you. You will easily find your style by understanding how what makes you easily understand. Seek the circumstances that you best learn at. Try to find places you can always put your skills into use. Remember practicing means you will not easily forget.

Metacognition requires that one uses their thinking to the extent of some control. Strategizing on ways a learning strategy that works best for a learner will help the learners in the long term — being able to see a task to the end until completion is also a metacognition skill. It takes a lot of skills to be able to identify yourself as a learner. Understanding your strengths and weaknesses, pushing on and accomplishing the whole learning process is an achievement on its own.

Students with extensive knowledge of metacognitive skills do very well in their studies. They can learn by themselves, utilize the right tools, and use their skills based on their respective expected areas. On the other hand, after they are done with school, they can use their metacognitive skills in the outside world. Metacognitive helps boost IQ, and therefore a person in the outside world can be very competent in handling groups in the workplace, take leadership positions and be perfect leaders because they can solve problems well without favor. Leadership positions require people who are well empowered with planning and monitoring skills. They are also good evaluators and can be able to evaluate situations in the workplace. Metacognitive skills will greatly help a leader is distributing roles to works, supervising and also help in conflict management. On the other hand, employee with metacognitive skills is very good at what they do because they know the strategies that will work for different tasks. They are self-regulated and therefore do not need much supervision.

People with metacognitive skills are well aware of their limitations and strengths and know exactly what tools to use in their respective tasks.

CHAPTER 9

THE BENEFITS OF VAGUS NERVE STIMULATION

Something I have seen time and time again, not only in myself, but in others, is how much vagal nerve stimulation can help your body. It's not just hocus pocus . . . this is all based on real science. Many studies have been done to prove how integral the vagus nerve is to so many functions in the body. When it's stimulated, we see major improvements in health, the reversal of unpleasant symptoms, and even the relief of many autoimmune diseases.

When we look at how well the vagus nerve works and how strong it is, we are looking at the vagal nerve tone, or how well your vagus nerve works. It's extremely important that your vagal tone is high if you want to stay healthy and be able to ward off diseases and stress. This can be done by stimulating or activating the vagus nerve. There are a number of ways to do just that, but first, you should understand more about the vagal tone.

Many factors can affect vagal tone and some people are more likely to have higher tone than others. For example, athletes and bodybuilders, as well as those who practice yoga, tend to have higher tone. Alcoholics, bedridden people, and those who don't exercise are at risk for lower vagal tone. It's also possible for you to have low vagal tone if your mother had low tone when pregnant with you. If she was stressed, angry, or anxious, it's likely that you were born with low vagal tone and may need to build it up.

Like bodybuilding, increasing your vagal tone means working out your vagus nerve. You need to keep activating it. How long should you do the activities given in this book? Fortunately, you don't need a long workout each day. You should aim for a total of 20 minutes or so per day. More is better, but as long as you are working on stimulating your vagus nerve daily, you are on the right track.

I suggest starting out by incorporating a few exercises into your daily routine. If you are rinsing your mouth, take the time to gargle a little longer. Showering? Sing or chant while you do so. It's fairly easy to add in a few little things and they all add up. The more you activate your vagus nerve, the more toned it will become and the more you'll notice yourself feeling better and stronger.

What is High Vagal Tone?

You want a high vagus nerve tone, since that means that your body is able to deal with stress very efficiently and can relax easily. It also means that your vagus nerve is better at regulating everything from digestion to blood sugar.

Essentially, your nervous system is honed and ready to control everything to keep your body functioning at its best. When you have high vagal tone, you'll be more mentally resilient and your body will be much healthier.

It's amazing to see the difference in your body when your vagal tone is high. I couldn't believe how much difference there was once I had spent the time activating my vagus nerve. It does take some time to see results, but you go from being stressed and anxious all the time to being calm and relaxed even after a difficult day. That was something that changed gradually, but when I looked back, I could see the huge difference between the before and after. A lot of people would benefit from being able to recover from a bad time rapidly.

Higher vagal tone means that you will feel less stress and anxiety and will be able to move on quickly from unpleasant events. If you know someone who seems to brush off even awful things that happen to them, it may be that they just have high vagal tone. This means their fight or flight response doesn't kick in for every little thing and they are able to process everything calmly.

When your vagus nerve is properly toned, you'll also experience fewer headaches, and overall improved health. One of the biggest reasons I found to aim for high vagal tone was the fact that it reduces inflammation. Since inflammation is the major cause of many autoimmune diseases and other health issues, keeping it at bay is a major reason to stimulate your vagus nerve.

What is Low Vagal Tone?

If your vagal tone is too low, you'll find that you get sick far more often than usual. Your immune system will function poorly, since it is receiving little stimulation from the vagus nerve and that means any illness, bacteria, or virus can take hold quickly and easily. This is often seen in those who are under a lot of stress or who feel anxious most of the time. They will also tend to be sicker overall and will catch every passing cold or flu.

Low vagal tone is also associated with depression and feeling down. This is something that greatly affected me when I was dealing with the aftermath of vagus nerve damage. It was a chore to get out of bed every day. While this was partly to do with the pain I was managing, it was also the ongoing depression that crowded into my brain. Many people will tell you that depression is simply the lack of serotonin in the brain and while this is partially true, the vagus nerve manages the release of hormones and neurotransmitters, so it is responsible for the release of serotonin. If you have low vagal tone, you'll find that depression sets in easily.

Depression has also been linked to poor diet, which affects gut health. We already know that gut health can be a big factor in how well the vagus nerve works, so it's logical that there would be a connection between depression and poor gut health, as well. Remember, it's all connected and everything in your body affects the other parts.

When your vagal tone is low, you will also deal with higher stress levels and anxiety. I'll go more into these areas later on, but having dealt with them personally, I can tell you that they are some of the more unpleasant aspects of low vagal tone. It can become almost impossible to move past a simple, stressful event. That's because your vagus nerve simply isn't able to work as well as it should, due to low tone.

If you do suffer from low vagal tone, there's still hope. Like a muscle, it can be improved by using it and stimulating it. The nervous system works best when it is being stimulated regularly and the vagus nerve is no different. In fact, there are plenty of ways to get your vagal tone up and it just requires knowing how to manipulate your nerves.

How to Measure Vagal Tone

Not sure if your vagus nerve tone is high or low? It is measured by looking at your heart rate. Everyone's heart speeds up slightly when they breathe in and becomes slightly slower when they breathe out. The difference between the two heart rates indicates just how toned your vagus nerve is. The bigger the difference, the higher your vagus tone is. If your body recovers quickly from just breathing, you know that you can recover quickly from other events, too. You should also check to see how fast your heart rate recovers from breathing in or out. High tone will result in a quick recovery, while low tone means the heart rate will lag slightly.

Your heart rate variation is the main way to test vagal tone, but there are other methods, as well. A simple way to check if your tone is high or low is to look at how you react to a stressful, yet harmless event. Do you dwell on it for the rest of the day and feel your anxiety spike every time you think about it? Or do you come up with a solution and move on to something else?

If you are able to calm your body automatically and move on with your day after a small, distressing event, your vagal tone is likely fairly high. However, if it haunts you for the rest of the day and maybe even overnight and into the next day, you may have low vagal tone.

Another method of checking is monitoring your breathing. It should be steady and not shallow or too fast. If you have the tendency to breathe too quickly and hyperventilate, you could have some issues with vagal tone. This is part of the reason you will find that breathing very deliberately and slowly will help you feel better.

Doctors may be able to check your vagal tone, as well, by measuring a combination of your breathing and heart rate. However, not all doctors are experienced with this method of diagnosing vagal tone and may not even be familiar with the term. It’s best to find someone who is already experienced in the area and can help you figure out if your vagus nerve is functioning correctly.

No matter how toned your vagus nerve is, you can always benefit from stimulating it. Even if you aren't able to officially diagnose low vagal tone, you can always start activating the nerve and chances are, you'll see an improvement in your symptoms.

The Effects of Vagus Nerve Stimulation

Scientists have discovered that it is possible to stimulate the vagus nerve with an electronic implant that you activate with a magnetic strip. It's something that has been used successfully in both animals and humans. Those who have ongoing, chronic conditions, reported amazing results when they stimulated their vagus nerve multiple times daily.

People who could barely get out of bed in the morning due to chronic pain and stiffness were able to dance and swim and walk again. It sounds like a miracle, but it's really just the body doing what it is supposed to. When the nervous system is fully functional, you should be able to feel great and be able to do things without feeling too much pain. Unfortunately, what has become the norm is due to vagus nerve damage or poor vagal tone, but this is rarely diagnosed correctly.

Perhaps the most famous of the participants in the electronic stimulation test was Maria Vrind. Maria was a gymnast in her younger days, but rheumatoid arthritis had destroyed her body and made it difficult for her to walk, much less enjoy the activities she used to. She went through many different medications, including cancer treatments that lowered her immune system. Since rheumatoid arthritis is caused by inflammation, lowering the efficiency of the immune system can help give relief, but it has other consequences. The cancer drugs can cause a number of side effects, including nausea and since your immune system is lowered, you will get sick very frequently.

Maria took part in a trial where an electrical implant was installed in her body and connected to the vagus nerve endings in her throat. From there, she had to stimulate the nerve multiple times a day. To her surprise, it only took a few weeks before she was able to return to gymnastics. Others in the trial had similar experiences and those who didn't experience a miracle cure still saw results and chose to keep the implant after the trial ended.

Even minor changes to the vagus nerve can cause impressive results. There are more and more studies being done now to prove that vagal stimulation is useful in the treatment of more diseases. We are constantly learning more about the mysterious nervous system, including the vagus nerve.

Doctors can now offer a medical implant to help treat epilepsy, depression, and autoimmune diseases. The implant just stimulates the vagus nerve on a regular basis, causing it to reduce inflammation and release the necessary hormones to keep our bodies functioning at peak performance.

While Maria and others in the trial used a medical device to electronically send signals to their vagus nerve, it isn't necessary to implant something in your body to stimulate the vagus nerve. You can do it at home, without any special instruments. It simply requires commitment, since it can take some time to see the effects. You need to be able to see it through, even when you don't notice any immediate changes.

For those who are interested in improving vagal tone without having to resort to an implant and electronic stimulation, this book is packed with ways to stimulate the vagus nerve naturally. You have many options and they are all simple enough to do at home. Some require more effort than others, but they are all useful in boosting your overall health and reducing unpleasant symptoms.

CHAPTER 10

ADRENALINE ADDICTION AND HIGH-RISK BEHAVIOR

Intent: To help warriors understand that a long-term, high-ops life tempo, along with combat experiences, leads to increased adrenaline, cortisol, and a natural high/euphoria.

Context: One of the challenges of being on deployment is that your body's homeostasis begins to acclimate to your surroundings. Thus, when in war, many unfortunately get attacked by things like RPGs or have to avoid things that are not natural in the civilian world, like IEDs. In Kandahar, we constantly got rocketed by the insurgency. The good news was that if you could hear the whizzing sound over your head, you knew it wasn't going to hit you because you could hear it. However, what you didn't know was whether there was another one on the way. And when you see the devastation that these rockets can cause to the body, ripping it to shreds, you quickly realize that you are not invincible. To mitigate this, you made sure that you hit the ground as soon as there was any indication of danger, whether that was the whizzing of rockets or an alarm indicating incoming fire. Your attention and being "on guard" was a direct result of wanting to stay alive.

This heightened sense of situational awareness and repeated exposure to stress in the AOR leaves a person in an elevated, hyped-up state, which is very similar to that of an adrenaline junkie. Yes, I said it, an adrenaline junkie. Adrenaline kept you alive when you were dodging Indirect Fire (IDF) and Direct Fire (DF). It allowed you to be sensitive to potential threats when you were risking your life on missions. It helped you cope with living in austere conditions while being away from your loved ones. It provided the energy boost necessary to keeping you effectively working 16-hour days during deployment, if not 24-hour days during combat missions. It was imperative to your survival. But you are now beginning to learn what happens to your body when it maintains elevated levels of adrenaline and cortisol over an extended period of time.

People wonder why they cannot sleep when they return home. It's because you are so used to this pace, this adrenaline, including a lack of sleep, and it's very hard to change those patterns back to baseline, especially when a person enjoys feeling very much alive. The rest of the world seems very boring once you've been "in the game." Sitting on the bench or even watching the world at its normal pace is an adrenaline junkie's nightmare. The loss of this thrilling and exciting natural drug produced by the adrenal glands is not something people want to lose. Many warriors actually deploy to a warzone repeatedly just to get the thrill of adrenaline back.

As a matter of fact, we had special ops guys who would come into the USO where I volunteered who played video games until all hours of the day and night. Instead of resting, calming down, and resetting their homeostasis, they and their buddies would stay amped up all the time on video games and power drinks. These same special ops guys actually beat the Black Ops video game within four hours of it coming out and walked out saying, "Well, that was easy."

ADRENALINE RUSH

The adrenaline rush is that surge of chemicals into your body that occurs under intense stress. Walter Cannon spoke of this in 1929 when he wrote about the various responses to stress: fight, flight, or freeze. Another name for adrenaline is **epinephrine**, and it's that intense and extremely fast chemical rush that occurs in the body when you are, for example, receiving incoming fire. It also happens when a loud noise goes off, especially when you least expect it. Controlled explosions are a little easier to take, because they usually announce them, and they are, by definition, supposed to be controlled. It's the **uncontrolled** explosions that really trigger our sympathetic nervous system. Just look at what happens when a car back fires near you.

Adrenaline has at least five benefits:

1. You often have a significant increase in strength (which

is why you hear of a mom who lifted a car off her child who was pinned underneath);

2. Diminished feelings of pain (which is why some people can get shot and keep going);
3. Elevated senses (such as seeing, hearing, feeling, and smelling things more intensely, which is also why people are triggered by certain smells that are emotionally attached to the triggering event);
4. Significant increase in energy (which can certainly help in times when a person's life is on the line).

Unfortunately, there are at least three downsides that accompany this elevated adrenaline-junkie lifestyle.

First, it destroys the body. It's like being on methamphetamine—all the time. The body needs rest, and it has to repair itself, but anyone who has been on a natural high really dislikes having to stop. Eventually, this person not only stops but also usually crashes, which, again, can be a good thing for people with sleeping problems, but it then only trains your body to go, go, go.

I can always recognize warriors with sleeping problems because they almost always have that look of exhaustion in the morning and are drinking some type of energy-boosting beverage or any drink that contains caffeine. They often get into a bad habit of using feeling threatened at night; then they can't sleep, and then they need an upper in the morning. You can see that when the body's normal cycle is interrupted by this drug-seeking behavior, it only complicates things. For example, the body's normal repair process, when interrupted, leaves you in an anxious, jittery state. You just feel on edge, and the slightest things irritate you. The body needs rest to bring back a more normal homeostasis, but this is often interrupted twofold: first by the environment of war and second by your decisions to stay elevated. Welcome to the adrenaline-addiction world.

Second, the mind has to have time to rest to make sense of the world and what you are experiencing. Part of the problem with living at a high adrenaline level or in chronically stressful environments is that areas of your brain responsible for memory (i.e., the hippocampus) and emotional processing (i.e., the amygdala) lose nerve cells (neurons) and connections between these cells (neuronal pathways). Brain imaging studies have shown actual physical changes in size, shape, and connectivity patterns of these pivotal structures. This can be significant because this affects your ability to regulate your emotions, to encode long-term memories, and to make new memories. If you wonder why you have difficulty understanding new concepts or remembering things, it could be that you are experiencing biological changes in your brain. You knew something was wrong, but you may not have known exactly the reasons why. But it gets better, and these changes can be reversed.

Third, you don't have to like adrenaline to be exposed to

chronically high levels. You may be thinking, "But I'm not an adrenaline junkie." The fact is that exposure to life-threatening situations for a prolonged period of time floods your body (and in turn, your brain) with adrenaline—whether you like it or not. Unfortunately, that's not where the story ends. It also begins to affect a stress hormone called cortisol. Cortisol is typically released in response to a threatening event or situation. Its job is to prepare the body to respond to the threat. However, in combat or disaster relief scenarios, the threat is prolonged for days, weeks, months, and, in some deployments, over a year. Our bodies are not meant to be flooded with cortisol for these extended, long periods of time. This chronic exposure causes the body to adjust to a new "normal," one in which cortisol does not ebb and flow as it does when we are in a normal, non-threatening environment. Instead, the body and brain are flooded with cortisol, leading to biological changes. These biological changes manifest themselves in symptoms that you are most likely familiar with, including memory problems, insomnia, weight gain, a weakened immune system, trouble coping, emotional outbursts, and adjustment issues.

Now let's just ask some very basic questions. Answer the following questions with a Yes or No.

Question	YES	NO

Do you have difficulty concentrating?		
Do you have difficulty remembering things?		
Do you find yourself irritable?		
Do you have difficulty sleeping?		
Have you gained weight since leaving the military?		
Do you find yourself getting sick more often than before?		

You may now be seeing the correlation between adrenaline, cortisol, and some of your problems. Much of this is biological. What does this mean for you? It means that your body is a magnificent vehicle that can adjust. And just as it adapted to develop life-saving strategies, it can be adjusted back with some of the tools and support in this workbook and through seeking out complementary treatment with a trusted, licensed therapist.

On a practical level, let's talk about what happens at night when you need the healthy systems to actually dream and not have nightmares. Nighttime is often a time when you run through the day's events and try to bring some sense of normalcy to it, but there is no "normal" in war. Trying to make sense of why people get killed, why certain decisions are being made, why we are there in the first place, missing home—you name it—is going to increase emotional responses and decrease ability to sleep. This process is interrupted mostly due to your elevated threat interpretation, which directly affects your amygdala, which, in turn, secretes more adrenaline into the bloodstream. This can then translate from normal, healthy dreams to nightmares, and this is the last thing a person wants to experience. As a matter of fact, they will do whatever they can to avoid nightmares, including purposeful sleep deprivation.

A direct correlation exists biologically between sleep deprivation and the effects of both adrenaline and cortisol. Unfortunately, through previous Stanford studies, we know that when someone goes without sleep long enough, the person can actually become psychotic. And by psychotic, we mean they can experience a break from objective reality. Do you want a combat veteran who is sleep-deprived, confused, and might become psychotic in the AOR when your life is on the line?

To be honest, you don't want an impulsive troop, especially if they have sociopathic tendencies. These are the men who take unnecessary risks that can put people's lives in danger. They are the hotheads who think they know better than everyone else. They are the first to jump up and take lead, even abandoning the mission's plans, including the commander's intent, just because they are looking for action. You can imagine this person coming back from deployment—highly anxious, sleep-deprived, angry, irritable, looking for a fight, engaging in high-risk behavior, feeling that everything is a threat, cannot get along with people, loses jobs, etc. Sound like anyone you know?

A great example of living like this is found in LTC Brad Holland. You may not know the name, but he is the guy who was infamous for living on the edge. As an adrenaline junkie, he enjoyed pushing things to the extreme. Unfortunately, Brad attempted a high-risk maneuver that pushed his B-52 bomber beyond the limits of its capacity to fly. In preparation for an air show, he lost airspeed in a high-banking maneuver, which created an unrecoverable crash and subsequent explosion. The event, caught on camera, is often used to illustrate how high-risk behavior can cost people their lives. His copilot, the only guy who would copilot with him, and two other crew members died that day.

COMING HOME

If any of these symptoms sound familiar to you, you may be an adrenaline junkie. Let's be clear: it has its benefits, but it also has its pitfalls. People often talk about going to substance abuse counseling, but when was the last time you ever heard of a debriefing on being an adrenaline addict? Let's take a little test to see how you would rate.

ADRENALINE ADDICTION TEST

Question	YES	NO
I drink power drinks or coffee or take stimulants to maintain energy.		
I seek out exciting, outdoor, high-risk behavior to keep me happy.		
I feel anxious/jittery.		
I wait until the last minute to do things and then rush to get them done.		
I feel that the rest of the world is boring.		
Others tell me that I overreact to situations, or I can sense they want to tell me but won't.		
I am always in the "on" position; "off" is best illustrated by exhaustion.		
I am easily startled by things.		
I find that when I'm not in control, things		

really bother me.		
I hardly ever feel a sense of calm, relaxation, or peace.		
I believe that losing is not an option and winning is correlated to effort; others don't try hard enough, and they easily frustrate me.		
I walk around a lot, and taking tests is a waste of my time.		
I am easily agitated by other people's driving habits.		
Being on time is not an option because I'm hardly ever on time.		
I am a firm believer that others simply want an easy life; they have no idea how vulnerable they are, and they would be easily killed by a terrorist.		
Finances are always a challenge because I spend money as soon as I get it.		
Focus and concentration are great as long as I'm being asked to focus on something I'm		

excited about; if not, you have my attention for about five minutes, and then I'm off in my head.		
Go, go, go is a motto; **hurry up and wait** is a stupid concept.		
When people are talking, I've already tuned them out.		
I sometimes have pressured speech because I have so much to say that I can't even get out what my brain is thinking.		
Racing thoughts occur at night when I'm trying to go to bed.		
I wonder if people think I'm crazy.		
Motorcycles, rock climbing, skydiving, and bungee jumping are things I would do in a heartbeat.		
My legs are jumping while taking this test.		
I have a very high sex drive.		
These are stupid questions; get on with it.		

Although this is not a standardized test, let's see how you did. Add up your **yes** answers and see the scoring chart below.

Scoring key

- 1–5: minimal adrenaline
- 6–10: moderate adrenaline
- 11 or higher: Let's just not go there, as your irritability may surface.

CONSEQUENCES

Unfortunately, people do not often change their behavior until consequences force them to. For example, you may not have sought treatment had it not been for loved ones or friends who basically indicated you needed help. They may not have known what to do, but they did know that something was wrong. Unfortunately, too many times we are thrown into a situation where we are forced to change because of consequences, which can be due to legal issues, marital/relationship issues, suicidal/homicidal ideation, mental health challenges, or a series of other reasons. Whatever the reason, we are glad you are reading this workbook.

The best way to change the addiction to adrenaline is to:

- **First, realize what it is doing to your body.** You have to be convinced that adrenaline and high-risk behavior are not good for you. Adrenaline causes heart palpitations, tachycardia (racing heart), arrhythmia (irregular heart beat), anxiety, panic attacks, headaches, tremors, hypertension, strokes, heart attacks, kidney damage, and acute pulmonary edema. None of these symptoms are enjoyable to live with, and over a long period of time, some can actually kill you. **Isn't it interesting that, once again, the same thing that kept you alive in a theater may eventually kill you if not treated properly?**

Between 5-10% of all visits to U.S. Emergency Departments are patients feeling as if they are having a heart attack. After thorough evaluation, they find out their heart is fine and that the effects of adrenaline are causing the anxiety/panic attacks. You won't die, but you have to learn how to control your anxiety.

Growing up, I was taught the art of moderation. The idea is that a person who is addicted to adrenaline is, unfortunately, off the chart regarding moderation. The consequences of this high adrenaline create many of the same symptoms we are trying to mitigate.

- **Second, adrenaline affects memory consolidation.** Adrenaline affects retrograde (past) memories to where they consolidate at a higher rate. During highly emotionally, stressful times, adrenaline creates a strong bond between intense emotional states, such as fear and memory consolidation. This is exactly why people with PTS(D) often remember their negative experiences in vivid detail. It is also common for people to try to use avoidance to not remember, but their own biology makes it almost impossible. For most of us, it doesn't take much, such as a particular smell or sound, to trigger us into a reflective moment called a flashback. We certainly don't teach ourselves to do this; it is a biological response that the brain has created. Remember that the brain's intent is to keep you alive, and it did; otherwise, you wouldn't be reading this. However, you are also no longer in a war zone, and it's time to get you back.

- **Third, we need to retrain your brain that not everything is a threat.** Since we were taught risk assessment, this is where we actually need to use it. What is important at this juncture is to understand that there is a clear biological reason why you interpret situations and people as a threat, even if they have no ill intent. This topic is so vital that we wrote a complete module to address it. "Module IX: Possibility vs. Probability" specifically focuses on threat assessment and risk mitigation.
- **Fourth, we will never forget.** I can only speculate that Adam and Eve had nightmares after Cain killed Abel. Do you think for one second that they could ever

forget what happened? NO! I'm sure they even blamed themselves and their parenting skills. Instead, we have to find a way to resolve our grief/loss and other issues, which is why we created the following modules: moral injury, survival guilt, and perspective.

- **Fifth, increasing one's resiliency factor and finding resolution is key.** Let me explain it this way. When Chris Kyle, the highly decorated American sniper, was asked if he ever had regrets for killing so many people, he could have said, "Well, I was brought up in church and taught to not kill. I also believe in the Ten Commandments. So, yes, these memories haunt me, and I can never get away from them. I see the faces of the people I killed, and at night I cannot forget them. I feel as if I will be in hell for what I did. I do not deserve forgiveness." But that is not what he said. He had resolved the killings in his mind, and, although paraphrased, his comment sounded something like this: "I only regret that I could not have killed more of our enemies so that more of our guys could have lived." Now that is a person who has resolved in his mind a potential internal conflict. In psychological terms, he is ego-syntonic with his thoughts, because, in the end, he was protecting our men by his actions. What our intent will be is to help you become ego-syntonic with your thoughts and actions to the point of resiliency and resolution.

CHAPTER 11

CHANGING MALADAPTIVE THINKING

Changing maladaptive thinking is an extension of psychology and one of its core principles. In this section we are going to discuss mainstream cognitive therapy.

Essentially this therapy holds that changes in maladaptive thinking will lead to changes in behavior. While this is true on the surface, there are other important factors to consider that are part of the reason why CBT is much more effective in and of itself than simple cognitive therapy is.

Cognitive therapy attacks cognitive distortions that are causing maladaptive behavior in a person's daily life. For example, the belief that everything a person does will fail is a cognitive distortion and needs to be challenged by the therapist.

Cognitive distortions and challenging the thinking however, are only the beginning of the process. The reason why CBT is so effective is because the main goal of CBT as we will see is all-inclusive and requires interaction and change by the patient.

The Main Goal Of Cognitive Behavioral Therapy

Cognitive distortions lead us into the importance of a complete therapy that takes into consideration the final goal of adaptive behavior, as well as the thoughts and feelings of the patient who seeks to normalize their behavior and interact successfully with society again.

This is what separates basic cognitive therapy from CBT; the ability to deal with the entire person and not just their thoughts. While no therapy is going to exclude the importance of behavior, CBT balances the importance of dealing with cognitive distortions along with behavior and allowing the two to work together in a way that also complements and supports positive feelings and emotions.

This makes CBT not only an effective therapy but one that can continue to grow with the person as they begin to appreciate better thoughts, better moods, better feelings and of course, better behavior.

Where behavior modification falls short, dealing effectively with moods and feelings on a cognitive level can then interact successfully with improved behavior.

This allows the therapist to not only function to address maladaptive behavior but to identify the causal links between cognitive distortions, acting out and the appearance of negative and/or maladaptive behavior.

Therapists are also free to teach patients the importance of dealing with all aspects of their humanity. Extending mental health therapy to people is a process that not only involves cognition but the ability to recognize what cognitive distortions are causing what pain in their lives.

For a person that has grown accustomed to cognitive distortions, it can take some time and even hard work to eventually get to the point to where their behavior begins to change effectively.

This has a very positive impact especially over time when dealing with people that are suffering from various degrees of mental illness.

Some of the more difficult and painful behaviors and thoughts can be challenged not immediately, but on a graduated scale that can be dealt with effectively by the patient. Therefore, CBT and its main goals are easily met, unlike some therapies that require useless repetition without much positive gain.

Effective Considerations For The Assessment

Once the assessment has been made, baselines have been taken, behavior modification suggested, as well as cognitive therapy introduced, we are now free to look at the larger picture because CBT involves many other aspects in a patient's life.

Treatment is best **not done in a vacuum** and should always involve people that are important to the patient. Even if the patient does not need to make all of the social criteria below part of his or her treatment, all of these aspects should be taken into consideration by the therapist and those that work on the treatment care plan:

- **Family & friends -** in order to preserve the integrity and privacy of the patient, the only family and friends involved should be the ones that are aware of the care plan. Here we also can involve people with just enough information to allow them to contribute their provided function. For example, a family member may only need to know that they wish to participate in a daily exercise to improve the person's mood and health, not that this item is actually ordered on a care plan.
- **Job/ workplace -** the only interaction that members at work should have with any patient should be in the form of stress reduction and should be done so carefully and cautiously through superiors. Changing job responsibilities slightly or moving the person to a new division that has less overall responsibility or a completely new way of doing work that would relieve prior anxieties of the patient could involve other peers. Despite most people's fears, this type of adjunct therapy is done frequently and quietly at most workplaces that offer the least restrictive environment for their workers.
- **Societal position -** the patient may have responsibilities in society such as sitting on a board, involvement with the local Chamber of Commerce, etc. Patients can temporarily step down or have another

family member take up responsibilities or reduce the amount of time devoted to such societal positions.

- **Personality** - the strength of personality is also important because this dictates exactly how the patient will interact with other people. Personality distortions, once they are corrected, can alter the way the person perceives reality and the way other people perceive this new aspect of an older or emerging personality.
- **Personal beliefs** - religious and/or ethical beliefs almost always impact behavior and therefore, should be a source of strength and not something that is restrictive in nature unless the person is emerging from an oppressive cult-like religion that is at the center of their disorders. Again, this is a thought process for the therapist and the patient.
- **Professional beliefs** - some patients hold very strong professional beliefs that can impact their behavior. For example, OCD people are often compelled to behave in repetitive manners that once cured, may seem to reduce their overall effectiveness and could impact their job performance.
- **Other considerations** - there are numerous other considerations that can impact diagnostics and/or suggested therapies that should be part of an overall baseline and screening. The key is to establish a

diagnostic snapshot that best allows the therapist to choose a course of action along with the patient who will also understand the importance is of managing the overall impact on their lives.

The key to understanding all of this is to realize that as therapy progresses people begin to change. The idea is to make the changes positive ones wherever possible and limit any type of negative impact on the person's overall life scheme.

Occasionally the importance of mental health far outweighs a person's current job, and after therapy, they may need to seek a different type or style of living contingent on the requirements for their new perspectives on health.

Intervention & Treatment Analysis

Both cognitive and behavioral therapy require an understanding as to the correct type of intervention and analysis for treatment based on events in someone's life.

Intervention and treatment analysis require that we understand the steps and considerations first and then determine the best approaches to this process.

Multiple treatments can and should be proposed based on:

- The best type of cognitive therapy.
- The best type of behavioral therapy.
- The best type of management of both the emotions and feelings during the other two therapies.

It is not the express goal of CBT to manage all aspects, all the time. Remember our main focus is on determining the best type of intervention first, after we take our baseline.

For example, Randy has constant panic attacks while he is in public and finds it difficult to talk to other people. The panic attacks happen anytime he is surrounded by people he does not know, and has to give an account of who he is or what he needs.

What most people would consider average everyday behavior, like going to the bank and withdrawing money, is an extremely awkward and difficult situation for Randy.

The therapist has proposed a form of systematic desensitization to teach him ways to learn how to deal with scenarios and situations of escalating stress.

This is a form of intervention and treatment analysis that the therapist has made. Such decisions should never be made in a vacuum, and require a firm baseline and understanding that this should be and is the best possible overall treatment.

Lacking sufficient background information, the beginning and/or intervention series requires several understandings:

- What information has been accrued during the baseline study that suggests the therapy or therapies that you wish to use are the best?
- What type of psychosocial focus should your therapy have, if any?

- Should the therapy or therapies that you choose involve scenarios that are painful yet necessary to help the potential patient through their disorders?
- What social tools can you use during an intervention and should the intervention be coupled with immediate therapy constructs? Why?
- What will be the impact of the therapy on the person's thinking, behavior, and feelings?
- Is it necessary to invoke discomfort during any of this process and how could this be avoided, if necessary? Should it be avoided at first?
- What are some of the top pieces of literature in the area and/or white papers suggesting based on your current situation as a therapist with the current patient that you have?
- Do you require the use of other professionals such as a drug addiction specialist, in order to reach a certain level of functioning to administer therapy?

All of these scenarios involve an understanding of exactly what you're going to do before you begin the use of any therapy, and if the intervention becomes confrontational or more passive in nature contingent on disorders.

The good news is that simply changing cognition can always be the first starting step before you begin to affect or impact behavior. Of course, this is contingent on a scenario in which behavior is not currently destructive and thus needs to be ceased immediately, such as hard-core alcoholism, drug abuse etc. Ultimately the term “intervention” need not be draconian in nature. Passive intervention can work just as well.

The Power Of CBT: Removal Of Erroneous Thinking

Therapists can now tap various behavioral models via the baseline information and use them to spot and reduce critical behaviors that are disturbing the client and causing breakdowns in thought reactive models.

In other words, now is the time for interventions based on assessment and to utilize top strategies with tools like thought stopping, passive confrontation and, cognitive modeling. In our next section, we will discuss in detail ways to deal with a variety of the top cognitive distortions that make people's lives significantly more difficult.

Understand that the main function of CBT is the removal of erroneous thinking. One of the best ways to attack this is to look for the most common cognitive distortions.

Erroneous thinking is the result of cognitive distortions plus possible misunderstandings based on feelings and emotions. The impact to the behavioral aspect is the end result of the cognitive distortions manifested into erroneous thinking that can also be linked with problematic feelings and emotions. Let us delve into this area of cognitive distortions and explain in detail the necessity for correcting erroneous thinking.

CHAPTER 12

FACING YOUR FEARS

For many people, a big part of their desire to deal with their mental health issues comes from the fact that their fears of objects, places, people or situations is starting to affect their life in an undeniable way. While it is normal to want to avoid things that you are afraid of, at a certain point avoidance actually starts to be counterproductive as it can make it much more difficult to realize that your fears are, generally speaking, not nearly as bad as you might think.

Practice exposure: In CBT, exposure is the process of gradually putting yourself into scenarios that trigger your fears in a controlled way to allow you to face them head on, leaving you less anxious and more in control as a result. Don't worry, when done properly, exposure doesn't ever actually put you in any danger and it is done in phases to ensure that it doesn't fully cause the trigger to activate in the moment.

What's especially useful when it comes to exposure is the fact that it allows each person who uses it to proceed at their own pace, building up confidence around trigger situations in their own way. Even better, you won't need to actively work to improve from encounter to encounter, the improvement will happen whether you focus on it or not, who knows, you may even end up enjoying whatever it is that you were previously afraid of. For example, if a person has a phobia when it comes to large bodies of water then they could start by standing in a swimming pool then slowly but surely immersing more and more of their body under water until they were eventually able to start taking swimming lessons and are some day able to swim in the ocean without issue.

If you have previously tried to shake yourself out of your fear and found that exposure did not work well for you then, it could be that you simply tried to rush the process more than your mind was willing, or able, to handle. Alternately, you may have simply not kept up the practice long enough to dull your fear to the point where it could no longer control you. Regardless, you don't necessarily need to believe that exposure therapy is going to work for you this time, you only need to start practicing it and keep it up for a long enough period of time to ensure you will start seeing results.

Seeing optimal results from exposure is possible, it is just going to take the proper planning, and plenty of patience. Remember, conquering your fears is a marathon, not a sprint, slow and steady wins the race.

Making a list: The first step to utilizing exposure properly is to know exactly what it is you are up against which means making a complete list of the objects, places, people and situations that you are afraid. This shouldn't be a general list either, it needs to be as granular as possible. For example, if you are afraid of dogs, your list may include petting a puppy, standing near a dog in someone's home, standing near a dog on a leash on the street, standing in an open space with a strange dog not on a leash, pictures of dogs, the sound of dogs barking etc. Each item on the list will then eventually become an action item that you will acclimate yourself to.

If you have multiple fears that are interacting with your life in a noticeable way, then you are going to want to make a separate list for each. While you will want to write all your lists at the same time in order to determine just what you are going to need to deal with, you are only going to want to focus on exposing yourself to one fear at a time. Don't kid yourself, kicking a fear, especially one that is deeply ingrained in your psyche, is a big task and you don't want to bite off more than you can chew, especially when you are just getting familiar with the process.

Organize your list: After you have created each of your lists, you are going to want to determine which you are going to want to tackle first. If the answer isn't clear up front, the best place to start is with a fear that is impacting you noticeably, but isn't necessarily the most intimidating on the list. This will provide you with a manageable goal to accomplish first to make sticking with the practice of exposure easier in the long-term, especially when you get to the more difficult fears on your list.

With your desired list chosen, the next thing you are going to want to do is put the items on the list in order starting with the most manageable and ending with the least manageable. Additionally, you are going to want to give each item a number on a scale between 1 (little or no fear) to 10 (crippling fear). With your list made, you will then want to start with the first, and least intimidating item. As you move through your list you will find that the things farther up it start to seem more and more manageable as you complete the tasks below it.

Once you have found a specific task to focus on, the next thing you are going to do is to make a list of all of the steps you would need to successfully take in order for you to successfully face your fear. For example, if you were dealing with a fear of social situations then eating a meal alone in a crowded restaurant may seem impossible, at first. However, it could then be broken down into steps that could be more easily accomplished such as:

- Go to a restaurant and get a coffee to go
- Have a coffee inside the restaurant but sit by exit on the patio
- Eat an appetizer at the restaurant and sit near the door
- Eat a salad at the restaurant and sit in the dining room
- Eat an entire meal at the restaurant on the patio near the exit
- Eat an entire meal at the restaurant in the dining room

You will then want to create a fear ladder for every one of your fears on your chosen list. Take note of each time a fear has an overlapping task, each of these will compress the overall amount of time required significantly and may even allow you to kill two or more fears with one fear ladder-based stone. Each ladder should include starter steps that you can do while only feeling a little bit of anxiety, before slowly scaling to scenarios that previously caused you moderate anxiety after between eight and 10 mild encounters. You will then want to up the ante to extreme anxiety situations, again, after another eight to 10 encounters. This is just an estimate, however, don't be afraid to take as small and gradual steps as you feel you need in order to find success.

Facing your fears: When you start utilizing exposure, the first thing you will need to keep in mind is that you want to push yourself past the point where you stop feeling comfortable, but not so far that your fear pushes you past the point of logical response. If the first thing you are afraid of isn't something you can do for a prolonged period of time, then ensure that you keep at it for a long enough period of time for the anxiety or fear about the activity to completely vanish. Alternately, you could try looping a shorter scenario by doing it several times in a row with only 10 or 15 minutes in between.

While the first or second time you attempt something, your physical response might be so intense that you can't react positively and have to retreat, once you are able to stand your ground you will find that your anxiety, while likely extremely high at first, will eventually subside. This isn't a question of if, it is a question of when, as remaining in an extremely anxious state consumes a lot of energy and it is simply not something the body can sustain indefinitely.

Once you are able to handle a situation to the point where your physical reaction begins to subside then you can rest easy, the hard part is over, the rest is simply inoculating yourself to the specifics of the situation and moving on to the next fear on your list. It is important to do everything in your power to set up scenarios that allow you to remain in as much control of the events as possible, to ensure that things go according to plan. The more in charge of the proceedings you feel when you start, the easier it will be for you to retain that feeling of control throughout.

CHAPTER 13

HEALING EXERCISES FOR BETTER SOCIAL FUNCTIONING

It is common for people to begin negotiating and bargaining in stressful situations. If stress continues, it is common to then become angry and frustrated. The next phase is to shut down. This is related to the more "automatic," or autonomic, nervous system. It is your sympathetic side that tells you to fight, freeze, or run. This is when your Vagus nerve is not activated. Blood flows into your muscles to help you survive. This means the blood moves away from your organs. The other system, your parasympathetic system, is all about relaxation. The idea of "rest and digest" being a nickname for the system is good, but it does not identify the importance of this function.

Your parasympathetic system rules your daily life. Your core functions are controlled by it. All things that come in or exit your body are governed mainly by your parasympathetic system. Long before humans evolved to be what they are today, and before most plant and animal matter existed, organisms had one cell, and were simply focused on bringing in nutrients and expelling waste. All of the evolution between then and today can be traced to these roots. Think about all the things your body does to remove waste and then bring in nutrients; breathing in and out, sweat, excrement and urine, menses, etc. All of these functions are primal and foundational actions necessary for survival. And they are all ruled by the parasympathetic system. This nervous system enlargers your blood vessels to flush out the skin and improve digestion. Birth, growing older, and healing from wounds are also part of this system.

During the process of evolution, beings began to develop legs and arms and other appendages. All designed to help that creature run from or to something else. Maybe the being now wanted to chase new food sources, or it needed to run from other creatures chasing it to eat it. This new development created a new nervous system in the body, the sympathetic nervous system. Now your blood moves less quickly, reserving it for later, and metabolism slows to conserve energy sources. It moves blood and other nutrients from the organs in the body and redirects it to muscles and these new limbs to encourage movement.

Your body activates the sympathetic system when it is stressed. But your body is not designed to stay in this stressful state. It is meant to enter it to either eliminate the threat or escape it. And when the moment passes, the body returns to the parasympathetic system's functioning. The problem is that now you do not live with real bears and dinosaurs chasing you, but with mental ones. Think about the job that you hate going to, the bad relationship you are suffering, the messaging on media channels about all the doom and destruction across the globe, etc. All of these provide stress to your body and keep it in this state because the stressors never seem to go away. There are many medical professionals who spend their days trying to get people to get out of this state. These professionals spend a lot of time talking about how important it is to "avoid" this sympathetic state. But in reality, you do not want to avoid it, just minimize it, or find a balance between the two.

Some doctors have discovered and published information about how to keep cardiac patients from relapsing or returning to the hospital. During their study and observation, patients were observed during cardiac rehabilitation. It is well known that operating in a high-stress, parasympathetic state for a long time can lead to the system eventually "wearing out." The functions necessary to keep your internal organs functioning begin to malfunction. Think about your heartbeat. You know your heart is beating fast because messages from your nerves triggered in the parasympathetic system; however, if those nerves become worn out, you may not recognize or be able to control your fast heart rate. But those that operated only in the parasympathetic state, not experiencing any stress for a long period of time, also had problems with the fading of their vital organ function, but in a different manner.

The evidence of this shows that an easy and peaceful body is not solely reliant upon a dominant parasympathetic system all the time. Think of it like cylinders; if you have two cylinders, but only fire from one, eventually that cylinder is going to burn out. There are consequences to "firing" from only one nervous system and not both. Like a car and its cylinders, if the body does this, it will begin to shut down and may even die. For organisms that still have one cell, the feigning of death is a survival technique. If that organism feared a situation, they appear to be dead. Some of those primitive responses include crying, attention-seeking, and silence. Think about the "silent treatment." It is a form of shutting down socially to alert the social threat of the other person. In a sense, you are "playing dead" until the threat is either extinguished or removed. But sometimes this response goes too far and ends up damaging your mind and/or body.

Friendships and rekindling old relationships are the "key" to helping cardiac patients during rehab. And it is a lesson that can easily be applied in your daily life, healthy heart or not.

This third system, the social nervous system, makes sense. The entire body and mind, including your nervous system, seeks balance inside and out. It wants to not only be harmonious in its internal functioning, but it also wants to feel harmonious with its surroundings. This is why, when your life is stressful and "stormy," you probably have a natural tendency or inclination to reach out to someone to find empathy. You want or even need to share with others because it is important for your survival to know that you are not alone and that what you are going through is not just a "you" thing or something that sets you apart from the rest.

With this information now in your "tool belt," you may feel like a fog has dissipated and you can finally see yourself and others more clearly now. Now that you know the social nervous system and the three systems and responses, you can recognize the stage a person is in. Not only does this help you, but it helps you see how other people are doing around you. Are they shutting down and "playing dead" because you or others have failed to acknowledge their needs? Or are they screaming for attention? Can you try and catch them when they are engaging their social nervous system and displaying the polyvagal theory in their facial expressions?

Your body and brain send out various energetic frequencies. Think about brain waves. These are like sound waves and are measurable frequencies. Researchers, such as Dr. Joe Dispenza, identified that infant brain waves are primal and connected to the development of the subconscious. During this time the subconscious is being developed and finalized with the important survival needs. It is developing a strategy to help you survive as you grow and later in life. When the infant reaches childhood, the brain waves and frequencies shift. They become more creative. Imagination and creative play, like turning an everyday object into a monster, dinosaur or horse. It is also why monsters live under the bed, etc.

These frequencies do not leave you when you become an adult, but often they become only active right before and just as you fall asleep. It is also common just when you wake up or when you are deep in meditation. These connections are very close to the subconscious. In these states, you have the ability to change the pattern of your neurology and "reprogram" what you learned as an infant and young child about survival among other things.

When you turn ten your brainwaves and energetic frequencies change again. Now they are more "mature" and follow a more rational approach. This change continues throughout adulthood. At this point the brain can identify the difference between different things, like the everyday object is not really a dinosaur and the shadow is just a shadow, not a monster. In addition, it provides the ability to rationalize emotions and situations. For example, you can find a rational reason why you should not deal with your emotions. But while you may convince your mind not to deal with it, eventually it will come out, and your body will respond in ways you cannot or do not want to control. You rationalize yourself into illness.

At this point, you have learned about the various stages of brain and energy waves, as well as the three nervous systems; social, sympathetic, and parasympathetic. You have also been introduced to the idea that the way adults respond to stressful situations, in particular, is due to the strategies they found which worked best for them when they were children. From a neuroscience point of view, this information is transformational. This information shows that the immune system, endocrine, and nervous system are all connected and working together inside you.

The concept is basic; if you are socially unable to cope with your stress, the body then begins to “fight, flight, or freeze.” This physiological state is not a place you want or should stay in long. If you do not cope with this threat or stress quickly, your body and mind start to fade. How you choose to interact with others includes the degree of interaction as well as the manner of contact. This determines the majority of your health. To find this balance and harmony, you need to do more than just meditate for 15 minutes every day by yourself or do a 30-minute relaxation yoga video by yourself. This is why the third system, the social nervous system, regulated largely by the Vagus nerve, supports your need to connect. Think about the importance of going to church on a Saturday or Sunday. You can pray at home but it is important to be together with others that support your view on spirituality. It is also why going to a fitness class is a far different outcome, especially on your happiness, than doing a program at the house by yourself. This means it is not about the actions physically, but about the connection socially. Studies at this stage people’s brain waves become calmer and more peaceful. And all of this knowledge then leads to a powerful change agent you can use in your future.

Anxiety, Social Situations, and the Vagus

Nerve

In Latin, the term "vagus" is a derivative of the word "vagabond." A vagabond is considered a wanderer, a person who travels is a loose fashion. While the Vagus nerve is not necessarily loose and meandering without purpose, it is still a nerve that travels around the body for a long time. It is like a river, the course of it moving from one place to the next, but with a direction and purpose. The purpose of the Vagus nerve is to communicate sensations to the brain. It is born in the brainbox, housed inside the spinal column at the base of your skull. It descends through your neck, wandering into the pharynx, larynx, esophagus, trachea, and bronchi. It branches into the lungs and heart, before coursing down into the stomach, pancreas, and liver. It communicates the messages from the brain to these places. But in addition, it listens to what is happening to the various organs and places that it passes by and sends that all back to the brain. This communication between a large majority of your body and your brain gets interesting.

All three systems have gas and brakes, essentially. And the messages sent to the body when the "gas pedal" is pushed determine how your brain responds to the environment and situation you are in. Think about when you are facing a bear. Your sympathetic system "floors the gas" to tell your body to move. This causes the other systems to slam on their brakes and let the sympathetic system drive for a bit. But the sympathetic system is like a young driver with a lot of road rage. It is wild and sometimes uncontrollable. It is not safe to let this system drive for a long time. But they sure are great at getting you away from trouble! The other two systems have their own drive and impact. For example, the parasympathetic kicks in when the danger is passed and the body can relax now. This system "takes the wheel" and begins slowing things down, getting back on the road, and following the road rules. To communicate in this manner, there are neurotransmitters spread throughout the body by the Vagus nerve. One such neurotransmitter, for example, is acetylcholine. This is designed to tell the heart to slow down and the bread pressure to lower in an effort to slow down the function of your other organs as well.

Most of this information has been shared before in this book; however, it is important that you remember how the Vagus nerve engages in several different functions in the body and how communication happens between organs and your brain. Your Vagus nerve is both highway and driver. Your organs and brain are simply the starting and ending points. Some of the functions that the Vagus nerve engages in or creates includes:

- Heartbeat regulation
- Breathing muscle movement and pace of breath
- Intestine and stomach muscle contractions to allow for

food digestion

- Digestion tract maintenance
- Stimulates relaxation after a stressful event to alert the body the danger has passed
- Tells the brain information gathered by your senses regarding the state of various vital organs.

CONCLUSION

Thank you for making it through to the end of this book. I hope you found something in this book that clicked for you; that you had the “ah ha!” moment that caused you to realize how much power you have. Anxiety and stress are tricky; they show up in daily life and have a sneaky way of making you believe that they are undefeatable. In many ways, your mind being your most powerful tool can also be your worst enemy, and it's all about training your brain to be on your side. Remember to be patient and kind to yourself. You are learning and growing. If it’s not troublesome, then it’s not making any positive changes in your progress. Remember that your healing process will take time, dedication, and a whole lot of faith in yourself.

Many of us know of pain as an undesirable sensation that arises from infections and injuries. However, pain is also an aftermath of certain disturbances in the normal functions of the brain and spinal cord. It can be assumed that the more stable a person’s mental state is, the more he or she has the potential to tolerate pain.

More importantly, people who experience anxiety should try to get to the root of their issues. Natural remedies should be seen treatment, not a cure. People should still work to find out what causes their anxiety, and take the steps necessary to reduce the amount of stress in their lives.

All the natural remedies suggested in this book can be helpful, always know that despite what you think, there are people that want to help you, that want to see you shine and come out on top. But remember, you always have to be there for yourself, even when nobody else is. You're capable, I know you are.

CPSIA information can be obtained
at www.ICGtesting.com
Printed in the USA
BVHW092249301120
594477BV00010B/1831

9 781801 323147